THE IRANIAN NUCLEAR CRISIS
Avoiding worst-case outcomes

MARK FITZPATRICK

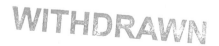
ADELPHI PAPER 398

11765180

The International Institute for Strategic Studies

Arundel House | 13–15 Arundel Street | Temple Place | London | WC2R 3DX | UK

ADELPHI PAPER 398

First published November 2008 by **Routledge**
4 Park Square, Milton Park, Abingdon, Oxon, OX14 4RN

for **The International Institute for Strategic Studies**
Arundel House, 13–15 Arundel Street, Temple Place, London, WC2R 3DX, UK
www.iiss.org

Simultaneously published in the USA and Canada by **Routledge**
270 Madison Ave., New York, NY 10016

Routledge is an imprint of Taylor & Francis, an Informa Business

© 2008 The International Institute for Strategic Studies

DIRECTOR-GENERAL AND CHIEF EXECUTIVE John Chipman
EDITOR Tim Huxley
MANAGER FOR EDITORIAL SERVICES Ayse Abdullah
ASSISTANT EDITOR Katharine Fletcher
PRODUCTION John Buck
COVER IMAGE AFP/Getty Images

Printed and bound in Great Britain by Bell & Bain Ltd, Thornliebank, Glasgow

British Library Cataloguing in Publication Data
A catalogue record for this book is available from the British Library

Library of Congress Cataloging in Publication Data
A catalogue record for this book is available from the Library of Congress

ISBN 978-0-415-46654-7
ISSN 0567-932X

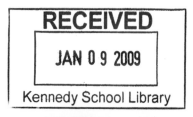

Contents

GLOSSARY

CTBT	Comprehensive Nuclear Test Ban Treaty
E3	United Kingdom, France, Germany (negotiating group)
E3+3	E3 plus China, Russia and the US
HEU	highly enriched uranium
IAEA	International Atomic Energy Agency
IRGC	Islamic Revolutionary Guard Corps (Iran)
LEU	low-enriched uranium
NIE	National Intelligence Estimate (US)
NPT	Nuclear Non-Proliferation Treaty
NSG	Nuclear Suppliers Group
PSI	Proliferation Security Initiative
UF$_6$	uranium hexafluoride
UNSCR	United Nations Security Council Resolution
WTO	World Trade Organisation

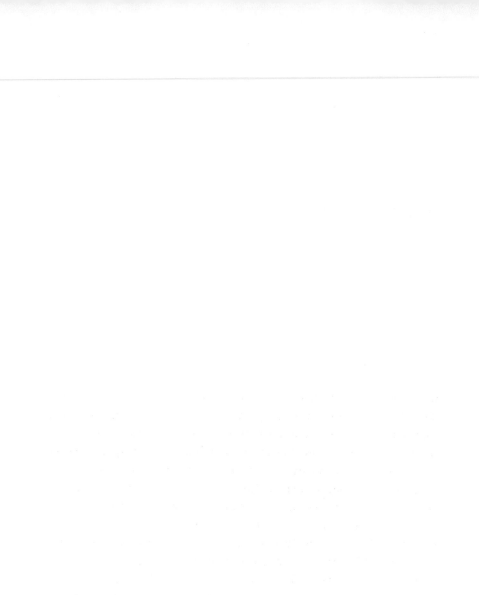

INTRODUCTION

Six years after the August 2002 exposure of Iran's uranium-enrichment and plutonium-production programmes prompted intense scrutiny, diplomatic enticements and financial coercion, the international community has failed to persuade Iran to stop work that will soon give it a latent nuclear-weapons capability. Although technical difficulties and limited components still may restrict the size and effectiveness of its programmes, Iran's ability to produce enriched uranium has become a fait accompli. Zero enrichment remains the goal of the major powers that have been engaged with Iran, although some, Russia and China in particular, realise it is no longer a credible objective. Recognising that an Iranian proliferation threat cannot be eliminated entirely, several private experts have suggested fall-back options designed to minimise the proliferation risks. If Iran is to have a fissile-material-production capability regardless, it is clearly better for it to be limited in scale and transparent in operation. Positing a need for such limitations presupposes, however, that enrichment within set limitations is acceptable. Indeed, for Iran ever to accept limitations on its nuclear programme, the rest of the world would surely have to accept the legitimacy of Iran's fuel-cycle facilities.

This monograph explores the options for building a barrier between a latent Iranian nuclear-weapons capability and an actual weapon, both in practice and in terms of perception. There is no guaranteed firewall between the peaceful nuclear activities permitted under the Nuclear Non-Proliferation Treaty (NPT) and weapons capabilities, but there are ways to make the gap between the two wider and more visible. The paper also addresses the policy question of whether accepting and granting legitimacy to an enrichment capability in Iran is the best way to minimise the risks, direct and indirect, stemming from Iran's nuclear programme. Even considering this option publicly carries some risk. Judging that current policy will continue to fail could become a self-fulfilling prophecy. If Iran believes that the West has a fallback plan, there is little reason for it to make any concessions before such a plan is offered. The potential gain to be had from later trading away the demand for zero enrichment is also lost. On the other hand, if policy has truly failed, then failure must be recognised for what it is, and adjustments made. Such adjustments will be better chosen if they have been carefully considered beforehand.

Operating on the assumption that zero enrichment is the only acceptable outcome, some commentators maintain that the only viable fallback option is military action aimed at disabling Iran's sensitive nuclear facilities.[1] This is not the 'second-best' option, however. It is the worst one. An increasing number of officials and analysts conclude that bombing Iran would be both ineffective and counter-productive.[2] Given the extent to which Iran has dispersed its nuclear activities, buried and hardened its facilities and kept many components out of sight of inspectors, air strikes would set back the enrichment programme for too short a period of time. Even if the underground enrichment plant at Natanz could be destroyed, it could probably be reconstituted within a few years, if not sooner, and in all probability no longer subject to inspection. In the aftermath of an unprovoked attack, Iran could be expected to withdraw from the NPT and engage the full resources of a unified nation in a determined nuclear-weapons-development programme. Bombing Iran's nuclear facilities would probably do more to spur than to delay the country's acquisition of nuclear weapons. Any gains that might be had from a bombing campaign would hardly be worth the risk of unintended consequences, such as terrorist attacks by Iranian surrogates and sympathisers on Coalition forces in Iraq and on private citizens and institutions throughout the world. Whether or not US forces participated in an attack on Iran, the US would be perceived to be involved. In the absence of a broadly recognised *casus belli*, the human suffering and economic losses stemming from such an attack would erode America's moral leadership and the solidarity of its alliances. The hardline Iranian government would garner more domestic and international support, severely weakening the international pressure on Iran's programme. An overstretched American military would become even more stressed to meet its goals in Afghanistan and elsewhere in the 'war on terror'.

Given these risks, it is well worth asking how the two worst-case outcomes of an Iran with the bomb and a bombed Iran can both be avoided. If military action would retard Iran's programme only by a few years or even months, after which the 'success' of such action would require its resumption, only this time with far less certainty about target location, can the same amount of time be bought with less problematic consequences? Unfortunately, time would appear to be on Iran's side as it advances its weapons capabilities. No country that has proceeded as far as Iran in nuclear-weapons development has failed to go on to weapons production.[3] There are no good options for dealing with Iran's nuclear challenge. As Harvard scholar Matthew Bunn puts it, the choice is between the 'least-bad' options. Which options these are should be determined on the basis of the expected risks to international security.[4]

CHAPTER ONE

Framing the Problem: Iran's Pursuit of Fissile Material

Iran's uranium enrichment: a unifying concern for the West

The problems and challenges presented by the Islamic Republic of Iran vary according to the geographical and political vantage point of the observer. To most Americans, as well as to the leaders of most of the Sunni Arab states that neighbour Iran, not to mention to Israel, the Islamic Republic presents a revolutionary, hegemonic, offensive threat. Many of Iran's policies and actions give grounds for offence: its military and financial support for Hizbullah, Hamas and Islamic Jihad; its abetting of civil strife in Iraq; its refusal to recognise Israel's right to exist and rejection of the Middle East peace process; its missile-development programme and its poor human-rights record have all made Iran something of a pariah. The 1979 occupation of the US embassy in Tehran and the Iranian state's connection with the bombings of US and French barracks in Beirut in 1983[1] also instilled deep resentment, among Americans in particular. Most Europeans, while viewing Iran's record in these areas as deplorable, see the country in less antagonistic terms.

It is Iran's quest for nuclear-weapons technology that enlists Europeans and many others in a shared threat perception. The fear that an unchecked Iran may soon have the potential to produce nuclear weapons unites nearly all on the Western political spectrum. For most Americans, a nuclear weapon in the hands of a terrorist-supporting enemy regime is the ultimate nightmare. Most other Western countries are more focused on the global non-proliferation regime and the damage to it that would be wreaked by a nuclear-armed Iran. If Tehran did not seek a nuclear-weapons capability, it is probable that there would be no transatlantic consensus on how to deal with Iran. In that scenario, however, Iran would also present far less of a problem. An end to Iranian enrichment and plutonium programmes would not resolve the deeper dispute between Iran and the United States. For that to be achieved, a far more comprehensive approach to the relationship would be required and, ultimately, a different government in Tehran. But an end to Iran's pursuit of capabilities to make fissile material would keep the Iran problem limited and manageable, restricted to that of a regional rogue, rather than a global menace.

The Iranian nuclear crisis centres on fissile material, not nuclear energy. From 2005, European offers to Iran, later joined by the US, Russia and China, reaffirmed Iran's right to nuclear energy and offered cooperation – including technical and financial assistance with state-of-the-art light-water-reactor technology – to help Iran to develop civilian nuclear power. This is in sharp contrast to Washington's pre-2005 opposition to all nuclear cooperation with Iran. Until US President George W. Bush and Russian President Vladimir Putin reached an accommodation in June 2005 about how Russia's support for the Bushehr nuclear reactor in Iran could be structured so as to reduce the proliferation dangers (through just-in-time fuel delivery, for example), the US consistently opposed Bushehr, on the grounds that it could provide a cover for work on more sensitive aspects of the fuel cycle and that the core of the reactor would contain enough plutonium for 100 weapons. But the new US acceptance of nuclear energy for Iran did not affect Iranian attitudes in any observable way. Iran simply changed its complaint about being denied the right to nuclear energy to an accusation that it was being deprived of the right to the nuclear fuel cycle.[2]

Seeking a weapons capability

Iranian officials insist that their country does not seek nuclear weapons. This claim is belied by the scale of the weapons development carried out prior to 2003, as revealed by documents under study by the International Atomic Energy Agency (IAEA).[3] However, the officials may be making a distinction between developing a weapons capability and taking the final step of building weapons. Iran's representatives are quick to point out that possession of nuclear weapons would undermine Iran's security by making it a sure target for US and Israeli attack and worldwide economic boycott, with the loss of the protection currently offered by

Russia and China. Iran also knows that overt development of nuclear weapons would stimulate similar efforts on the part of its Arab Sunni neighbours, thereby negating its conventional strategic advantage.[4] In addition, Iranians point out that in August 2005 Supreme Leader Ayatollah Sayyid Ali Khamenei issued a fatwa against the development, production, stockpiling and use of nuclear weapons. Fatwas may be changed on the grounds of new circumstances, but, given the pervasive religiosity of the regime, it is unlikely that Iran's supreme leader would be secretly endorsing military activity in explicit contradiction of his own religious edict.

Viewed from the outside, therefore, Iranian intentions are unclear. In any case, Iran's leaders do not yet need to make a decision about whether to produce nuclear weapons. They can wait until after the fissile material is produced to decide if and when to develop the physics package needed for a weapon. French strategic analyst Bruno Tertrais draws an instructive parallel with France, which reached the threshold of weapons capability in 1958 without ever having taken a clear and firm decision to produce nuclear weapons.[5] What Iran has certainly decided is to acquire the technical capability to produce fissile material. Its nuclear hedging strategy is designed to bring the country right up to the threshold of a break-out capability while remaining within the legal limits of the NPT. This goal commands strong support within Iran's political elite and the country at large. A difference between pragmatic conservatives and hardliners, however, is that the former are willing to negotiate on the time frame for developing a weapons capability, while President Mahmoud Ahmadinejad and his coterie will brook no delay.[6]

The November 2007 US National Intelligence Estimate (NIE), an unclassified version of which was released on 3 December, concluded that Iran had stopped explicit nuclear-weaponisation activity four years earlier. The NIE also concluded that Iran's uranium-enrichment programme gives it the option of developing nuclear weapons in the future. Producing fissile material – either highly enriched uranium (HEU) or weapons-usable plutonium – is the hardest part of developing a nuclear bomb. The weapons-design work that the NIE judges Iran to have halted in 2003 can be picked up again at some future date. Meanwhile, if its uranium-enrichment programme continues unabated, Iran will be in a better position to produce a bomb quickly if it so decides. Work is also proceeding apace on the third main ingredient: a range of missile systems to serve as delivery vehicles.

Iran's motives

It is not difficult to understand Iran's motives for seeking a nuclear-weapons capability. Iran launched its uranium-enrichment programme in the mid 1980s during the war with Iraq, after being attacked with chemical weapons. This decision, which was taken for a number of reasons, overturned the leadership's original opposition, based on moral grounds, to the shah's nuclear programme. Iranians argue that Saddam Hussein would not have dared to start the war or use chemical weapons if Iran had possessed a nuclear capability. It is also often remarked that Iran inhabits a dangerous region, with four neighbours possessing nuclear weapons and a domineering superpower with troops positioned to its east in Afghanistan and to its west in Iraq, and with naval forces off its coast to the south.

Leaving aside the US factor for the moment, however, the relevance of the proximity of nuclear-armed countries has far more to do with national pride than national security. Although Iraqi missile and chemical-weapons attacks were certainly a motivating factor behind the resumption of the enrichment programme in the 1980s, Iran today seeks a nuclear-weapons capability not so much for deterrence as for the prestige that possession of such advanced technologies bestows. Pursuit of sensitive technologies is an emotive assertion of sovereignty for a nation with still-vibrant memories of national humiliation and dependence on major powers. Iran characterises its enrichment programme as a basic national right, central to Iranian sovereignty and nationhood. Invested with the symbolism of scientific progress and national power, the nuclear programme has widespread domestic backing. Indeed, the programme partly functions to legitimise a regime that has otherwise lost popular support.

Iran's regional leadership aspirations are another driver: possession of a nuclear-weapons capability is seen as conferring the major-power status that Iran seeks. The deterrence factor too cannot be denied. Pronouncements assigning Iran to the 'axis of evil', a policy of 'preventive deterrence' and loose talk of regime change on the part of the US have undoubtedly motivated the Iranian leadership to develop the ability to resist coercive measures. To the extent that the US and Israel present a direct military threat, however, it is the result of circular causality. The only reason for attacking Iran would be to pre-empt a nuclear threat.

The military purpose of Iran's enrichment activities can be deduced from three sets of factors: the clandestine history of the programme; the military connections to it; and its economic illogic.[7]

Secrecy and deception

According to statements made to the IAEA, shortly after Iran launched its uranium-enrichment programme in the mid 1980s, it contacted the nuclear-black-market network led by Pakistani metallurgist Abdul Qadeer Khan for the basic technology and a starter set for gas-centrifuge enrichment.[8] The Khan network was in the business of nuclear weapons, not civilian nuclear energy. Iran kept the Natanz enrichment plant and a heavy-water-moderated research-reactor construction site at Arak hidden until August 2002, when they were revealed by an exile group (which made public what Western intelligence agencies already knew but could not disclose without risk to intelligence sources and methods). Iran rationalises that under its IAEA safeguards agreement at the time, it had no legal obligation to report Natanz or Arak to the agency until six months before the introduction of nuclear material into those plants. But it did have a legal obligation to report the import and use of nuclear material in general, and the facilities (at the Kalaye site outside Tehran and elsewhere) in which it was used. When IAEA officials were finally able in 2003 to visit Natanz, Kalaye and other facilities and to investigate Iran's programme, they documented 14 different ways in which Iran had systematically violated its safeguards agreement over an 18-year period.[9] Iran then repeatedly misled inspectors, and changed its story when confronted with evidence that contradicted its statements.

It was because of the violations uncovered in 2003 that, in September 2005, the IAEA Board of Governors found Iran to be in non-compliance with its safeguards obligations.[10] A non-compliance finding had been put off for as long as Iran suspended its enrichment activity, which it did, partially and fitfully, until August 2005. The safeguards violations undercut Iran's claim that it has a right to enrichment and reprocessing under the NPT. Article IV of the NPT makes the right to nuclear energy for peaceful purposes conditional on fulfilment of non-proliferation obligations. Iran's legal case for the right to enrichment was further undermined by UN Security Council Resolution 1696, passed 14 to 1 on 31 July 2006.[11] That resolution and the four more that followed between December 2006 to September 2008 make it mandatory under Chapter VII of the UN Charter for Iran to suspend all enrichment-related and reprocessing activities. By disregarding this demand, Iran is in continuous breach of international law. This will remain the case even if it fully adheres to its safeguards agreement, unless it suspends enrichment or the Security Council adopts a superseding resolution.

Military connections and alleged weaponisation studies

At least ten signs of military involvement in various aspects of Iran's nuclear programme and nuclear-weapons-related procurement and research have been enumerated in IAEA reports.[12] In February 2008, the IAEA judged that Iran's answers to questions about two of these areas (polonium-210 experiments and the management of the Gchine uranium mine by a suspected military front company) were consistent with the agency's findings. While not a total exoneration, this closed the file on these questions for the time being. The agency also assessed that answers regarding two other issues (the procurement activities of a former head of Iran's Physics Research Centre and radiation contamination of equipment at a technical university) were 'not inconsistent' with its findings.[13] This phrase indicates that the IAEA had a lower level of confidence that these answers were complete, and that it had not yet been able to verify all the answers to its questions. Another military connection can be seen in a 15-page document that Iran received from the Khan network in 1987 describing the procedures for the reconversion and casting of uranium metal into hemispheres, which IAEA Director General Mohamed ElBaradei has described as 'related to the fabrication of nuclear weapons components'.[14] Iran insists that it received this document on the initiative of the network. In September 2008, the IAEA was still seeking further information from Iran about the circumstances of its acquisition of the document.

The most damning evidence of military connections to Iran's nuclear programme came from the thousands of documents stored on the hard drive of a laptop computer that was turned over to a US embassy in the Middle East in 2004 by a walk-in defector,[15] apparently taken without the knowledge of its owner. Many of the documents related to an alleged nuclear-weapons-development effort known as 'Project 111', apparently under the control of the Iranian military and directed by Mohsen Fakhrizadeh, a nuclear engineer who formerly headed the Physics Research Centre and is reportedly a brigadier-general in the Islamic Revolutionary Guard Corps (IRGC). The information included references to a 'Green Salt Project' for the conversion of uranium yellowcake into uranium tetrafluoride, one of the steps in the enrichment process. The hard drive also held designs for a ballistic-missile re-entry vehicle to carry an object that had all the attributes of a nuclear weapon. Other documents on the laptop contained scientific notes highly suggestive of triggers to compress HEU spheres into a critical mass for an atomic explosion, as well as sophisticated drawings for a 400-metre-deep shaft that appeared designed for an underground nuclear test. The most recent documents on the computer were dated 2004, shortly after the US NIE concluded that Iran had stopped explicit weaponisation work.

Despite Iran's efforts in August 2007 to limit the questions it would have to answer by agreeing with the IAEA a 'work plan'[16] for addressing outstanding questions, agency reports of May and September 2008 indicated that the evidence about military connections and weapons purposes continued to expand. Among this evidence was a letter written in 2006 by the chairman of Iran's Expediency Council (an important adjudicatory body) making reference to the possible acquisition of nuclear weapons,[17] and a document describing 'experimentation undertaken with a complex multipoint initiation system to detonate a substantial amount of high explosive in hemispherical geometry'[18] – a fitting description of the use of explosives in a nuclear weapon. In September, the agency stated that it had received information that this experimentation may have drawn on foreign expertise, which the *New York Times* later reported to be a Russian scientist believed to be working alone.[19] At the same time, the Iranian government was still refusing to provide satisfactory answers to questions about the alleged nuclear-weaponisation studies. Nor had it allowed the agency to interview Fakhrizadeh or other individuals said to be associated with the alleged studies.[20]

Missiles
Iran's ballistic-missile programme magnifies the threat. With technological help from North Korea, Iran fields a *Shahab*-3 missile whose 1,300 kilometre range encompasses Israel, Turkey and Saudi Arabia. The *Shahab*-3 has the payload capacity (approximately one tonne) and the airframe diameter (greater than 1.2m) necessary to carry a nuclear warhead. If Tehran were to develop and manufacture a nuclear weapon, the *Shahab*-3 or its variant, the *Shahab*-3M, would be the preferred delivery vehicle. In September 2007, Iran showed off a longer-range missile, labelled *Ghadr*-1, which had a 1,800km range, and in July 2008, it tested a version of the *Shahab*-3, sometimes called a *Shahab*-4, that had a claimed range of 2,000km. Using Soviet technology acquired via North Korea, Iran is also understood to be working on a 2,500km-range missile, known variously as a *Shahab*-5 or BM-25, which could reach many parts of Europe.[21] Work on a two-stage *Safir* satellite launch vehicle further contributes to Iran's missile capabilities.[22] There are also unconfirmed reports that Iran seeks to build *Shahab*-6 medium-range missiles[23] with ranges of 4,500km to 5,500 km, which would put most European cities, including London (4,400km from Tehran), within its reach. The limited accuracy of Iranian ballistic

missiles makes them primarily valuable for delivery of weapons of mass destruction. In addition, Ukraine reported in 2005 that Iran had acquired 12 old X-55 cruise missiles from a Ukrainian black-market dealer four years earlier.[24] The X-55 (also known as a Kh-55) was designed to carry nuclear weapons and has a 3,000km range.

Economic illogic of indigenous enrichment

The economic rationale that Iran has put forward for seeking indigenous uranium enrichment is flawed in three respects. Firstly, Iran's arguments for enrichment are predicated on the need for self-sufficiency in fuel supply, but its domestic uranium reserves are insufficient for the number of reactors it plans to build. It would thus need to import uranium in any case. Secondly, given the ready availability of enriched uranium fuel on the international market, indigenous enrichment does not make economic sense for states that have fewer than five to ten reactors.[25] It is far cheaper for Iran to buy enriched uranium fuel, as it has done already for the Bushehr reactor. Thirdly, Iran's insistence that it needs to produce its own low-enriched uranium (LEU) in order to ensure a supply of fuel for the billion-dollar Bushehr reactor and future planned nuclear power plants is disingenuous. Once Russia had delivered its first fuel load for Bushehr in the winter of 2007–8, Tehran began insisting that it now needed to produce its own fuel for a 300MW light-water reactor under construction in the town of Darkhovin near the Kuwait border. Whether Iran could build a safe power reactor on its own is, furthermore, open to question, and in September 2008, Iran had not yet acceded to the IAEA's request for preliminary design information for the Darkhovin plant. In any case, there are many other ways of guaranteeing an LEU fuel supply, including by taking advantage of one or more of the dozen proposals to ensure LEU supplies that have been tabled in the past couple of years by states and international organisations. These include a Nuclear Threat Initiative project for a fuel bank under IAEA auspices, which in October 2008 was nearing its funding target of $150 million, and a Russian plan to donate $300m-worth of LEU produced by its international enrichment facility at Angarsk in Siberia for guaranteed supply to any country meeting criteria determined by the IAEA.[26]

If Iran is really concerned about disruption of reactor-fuel supply, it should focus not on uranium enrichment but on fuel fabrication. LEU is commonly referred to as reactor fuel, but this shorthand skips over the sophisticated work required to fabricate the actual fuel. The LEU gas must be reconverted to dioxide powder, which is then pressed into small pellets.

The pellets are then sintered and stacked in long tubes, known as rods, surrounded by leakproof zirconium-alloy cladding and grouped in cage-like fuel assemblies. There are many suppliers of LEU from whom Iran could choose, but there are only two potential suppliers of fuel assemblies for the Bushehr reactor. Fuel-assembly designs are highly specific to reactor type. Using fuel assemblies made elsewhere that have not been certified by the reactor builder could result in damage to the power plant and would be a contract violation entailing certain voiding of the supplier's liability. Fuel fabrication is not a proliferation-sensitive technology, so in principle there should be no international opposition to Iran building its own fabrication plant, although Russia would need to be persuaded to cooperate in sharing the reactor-core specifications so that the fuel could be certified.

Sensitive technologies

Uranium enrichment is the process of increasing the concentration of radioactive U-235 isotopes from the average 0.7% found in uranium in nature either to 3.5–5% to make fuel for reactors or to above 90% for nuclear weapons. Gas centrifuges are the enrichment technology of choice today, in Iran and elsewhere, but several other technologies are also possible, including atomic vapour laser isotope separation (AVLIS), which Iran experimented with between 1991 and 2003. Centrifuges spin at supersonic speeds to separate out U-235 isotopes from heavier isotopes using centrifugal force. The P-1 ('Pakistan first-generation') centrifuge that is the mainstay of Iran's enrichment programme spins at 800–900 miles per hour. It is based on technology developed in the 1960s by international enrichment company Urenco, which A.Q. Khan stole from a Urenco subsidiary in the Netherlands for Pakistan's nuclear-weapons programme and began selling to Iran from at least as early as 1987. Khan also provided Iran with the technology for P-2 centrifuges, Urenco inventions from the 1970s that are more than twice as powerful as P-1s.

Although not restricted by the NPT, uranium enrichment and plutonium reprocessing (the separation of weapons-usable plutonium from reactor spent fuel) are considered sensitive technologies because in addition to their civilian purposes, they can be put to weapons use. More than three decades ago, influential US strategist Albert Wohlstetter warned of the proliferation risk posed by countries that, despite abiding by their NPT obligations, were coming close to possessing nuclear weapons by developing these sensitive technologies.[27] Uranium enrichment is the dual-use nuclear technology of greatest current concern with regard to Iran because it is Tehran's preferred path. However, the heavy-water-production facility and heavy-water-moderated research reactor under construction at Arak could give Iran an alternative plutonium path to nuclear weapons, if it also acquired a facility to separate, or reprocess, the plutonium from the reactor's spent fuel. Like enrichment, plutonium-separation technology became available on the black market in the 1980s.[28] Similar to Pakistan's Khushab heavy-water-moderated research reactor, the 40-megawatt Arak plant would be ideal for producing weapons-grade plutonium. It will be of growing concern as it nears completion, scheduled for 2009 but likely to be delayed for a few years.

In shorthand, enrichment and reprocessing are sometimes referred to as 'the fuel cycle', because with these two technologies a state can complete the full nuclear fuel cycle: from uranium mining and milling to gaseous conversion, through fuel enrichment and irradiation to spent-fuel management and reprocessing. Although the Iranians are not known currently to be working on any reprocessing activity,[29] since 2006, all IAEA resolutions and UN Security Council resolutions have stubbornly called on Iran to suspend both 'enrichment-related and reprocessing' activities. 'Enrichment-related' means both enrichment and uranium conversion (the chemical conversion of powdered uranium yellowcake to gaseous uranium hexafluoride (UF_6)), as well as the manufacturing of centrifuge components. In the calls for suspension, these activities were lumped together with reprocessing on the grounds that, along with heavy-water-related activities, they were all proliferation-sensitive. It would be more logical and accurate for the resolutions to call on Iran to suspend enrichment-related activities and to abstain from reprocessing. Alternatively, the resolutions could have simply demanded that Iran suspend all 'sensitive' fuel-cycle activity. But once the IAEA Board members reached a compromise on the language in 2006, diplomatic stasis and a desire not to break the consensus stifled any impulse to fix the language. The issue is ripe for revisiting in future negotiations. Iran says it has no plans to develop a reprocessing capability, and has said that it will commit to refraining from building reprocessing facilities if its enrichment programme is accepted.[30]

Although enrichment-related activity was the political trigger that sent the Iranian nuclear issue to the Security Council in 2006 and prompted the sanctions resolutions that followed, it was not in itself the legal rationale for the decision of the IAEA Board of Governors to report the issue to the Security Council that year. The legal basis for reporting Iran was twofold: that Iran's failure to comply with its safeguards reporting requirements over an extended period constituted safeguards non-compliance under Article XII.C of the agency's statute; and that Iran's history of concealment of enrichment-related and other nuclear activities, and the resulting absence of confidence that its programme was exclusively for peaceful purposes, gave rise to questions within the competence of the Security Council, thus requiring a report to the Council under Article III.B.4 of the agency's statute.[31]

Western states deemed it important to include the second rationale in the September 2005 IAEA Board resolution that established the legal basis for reporting Iran to the Security Council. This was in case Iran took action to remedy the causes of the non-compliance finding, which could put Security Council consideration on a tenuous legal footing. With the second legal element, even if Iran retrospectively fulfilled all of its safeguards reporting requirements and addressed all the IAEA's outstanding questions about those reporting failures, there would still be a basis for Security Council action – the ongoing lack of confidence that Iran's nuclear programme was for peaceful purposes.

Would coming clean on past activities be enough?
Not all Security Council members agreed. Most notably, Russia indicated in autumn 2007 that if Iran answered all the IAEA's questions and explained past activities that had given rise to suspicion, it would not support another sanctions resolution.[32] Such a scenario would be problematic, because Iran's coming clean on past activities would not allay fears that its continuing enrichment activities were laying the foundation for a weapons programme. Those fears are not based solely or even primarily on Iran's safeguards violations. Although the violations buttressed the Western case, concerns began longer ago, when Iran first began seeking dual-use facilities.

To achieve a nuclear break-out capability, Iran's best strategy would be to cooperate fully with the IAEA in order to restore as much confidence as it could and then to proceed with a safeguarded but unfettered enrichment plant. In agreeing in 2007 on a work plan for addressing the IAEA's outstanding questions, Iran appeared to be following such a strategy, and, by February 2008, the IAEA report was able to say that the 'one major remaining issue' was the 'alleged studies on the green salt project, high explosives testing and the missile re-entry vehicle'[33] (i.e., Project 111). It was perhaps generous to call this the 'one' remaining issue, in view of its damning substance and the multiplicity of evidence about the project, later detailed in the IAEA's May 2008 report. Satisfactorily addressing questions about the alleged studies is politically unpalatable for Tehran because it would require admitting to past weapons-development work and risk a new round of condemnations and sanctions, unless such an admission were to be pre-emptively forgiven by the Security Council. Iran insists that it has addressed all aspects of the work plan[34] and that it should therefore be taken off the Security Council's agenda and its status in the IAEA returned to that of a country following normal safeguards.

The Additional Protocol: necessary, but not sufficient
ElBaradei has repeatedly emphasised[35] that the IAEA will not be able to provide assurances about the absence of undeclared material and activities from Iran unless Iran addresses the outstanding questions and implements the Additional Protocol. This document, agreed upon by the IAEA Board of Governors in 1997, gives the IAEA expanded rights of access to information and sites and was, at the time of writing, in force in 82 states. It would be incorrect, however, to draw the conclusion that if Iran took these steps, a clean bill of health would be forthcoming. The Additional Protocol would help to provide transparency, but it is important to recognise the limitations of this verification measure. It does not provide for inspector access 'anytime, anywhere to all data, places and people',[36] and inspectors still would not be able to detect undeclared activity without prior information about the location of the activity. The Additional Protocol gives the IAEA Secretariat a basis for providing credible assurances about the absence of undeclared nuclear material and activities. But the Secretariat cannot give these assurances until the state in question has satisfactorily resolved questions and anomalies that have arisen in the verification process. As long as one IAEA member state provides information that raises legitimate questions, the Secretariat will not be on solid grounds to provide full assurances. In other words, Iran will not be in the clear until it gives no further reason to question its non-proliferation bona fides and can show a sustained record of compliance and transparency.

The question is whether even a fully compliant, fully transparent Iran could be trusted with enrichment. Given the apparent military purpose of its programme, there is reason to fear that Iran might break out of the NPT and use a stockpile of LEU to quickly produce HEU for weapons purposes. This concern is not diminished by the fact that the IAEA has never found any evidence of diversion. As explained in the next chapter, diversion is the least of the potential proliferation risks. It is far more difficult to guard against clandestine replication of facilities, and IAEA inspections are no defence at all against break-out. The only guaranteed prevention of such a scenario is for there to be no enrichment activity at all.

No enrichment: a consistent transatlantic objective

Insistence that Iran not enrich uranium has been a constant central theme of transatlantic policy towards Iran. The first IAEA Board of Governors action on the subject came in June 2003: a request that Iran, as a confidence-building measure, refrain from introducing nuclear material into the centrifuge cascades at the pilot enrichment plant at Natanz.[37] This request, which took the form of a chairman's summary rather than a resolution, followed a report from the IAEA Secretariat that Iran was about to take this step and that it had earlier failed to meet reporting obligations laid out in its safeguards agreement.[38] The US argued that this was grounds for a finding of safeguards non-compliance, but other Board members argued that Iran should first be given time to correct its reporting failures. The United Kingdom, France and Germany (the 'E3', an abbreviation that came to be preferred over 'EU3' because it did not imply that they were representing the EU) then began a diplomatic engagement effort designed to divert Iran from its path using European economic leverage. In an August 2003 letter to Iranian Foreign Minister Kamal Kharrazi, Foreign Ministers Jack Straw, Dominique de Villepin and Joschka Fischer urged Iran to, inter alia, 'cease its development of facilities which would give it the capability to produce fissile material, including any enrichment or reprocessing capability'.[39] Iran had by this point already begun introducing UF_6 into a small number of centrifuges in defiance of the Board's June call not to do so. In order to forestall any Board moves to send the issue to the Security Council, however, Iran voluntarily agreed, in a joint statement at the end of a visit to Tehran from the E3 foreign ministers in October, to suspend all uranium enrichment and reprocessing activities 'as agreed by the IAEA'.[40]

In talks leading up to the October 2003 agreement, the Iranian negotiating team had insisted that no joint statement could cite 'permanent cessation' as the E3 goal. The agreement therefore used instead the euphemism of 'satisfactory assurances' to denote the objective of ongoing negotiations, which the E3 ministers made clear to the Iranians meant permanent cessation.[41] Ambiguity about what the suspension covered caused repeated problems in the ensuing negotiations. In November 2003, the IAEA Secretariat informed the Board that Iran had decided to suspend all activities at the Natanz site, not to produce feed material (UF_6) for enrichment and not to import enrichment-related items. Iran subsequently said that the suspension did not include the making of centrifuge components under existing contracts or the production of feed material. By June 2004, Iran had restarted the manufacture of UF_6. Disagreements over the scope of the suspension continued until November 2004, when Iran agreed to a new deal with the E3 spelling out the suspension conditions in detail. Signed in Paris, this agreement said that suspension would continue while negotiations on a long-term agreement were under way, and that the long-term arrangements that would come out of those negotiations would 'provide objective guarantees that Iran's nuclear programme [was] exclusively for peaceful purposes'.[42]

The E3 negotiations with Iran centred – and eventually foundered – on the meaning of 'objective guarantees'. For the Europeans, this was another euphemism for complete and permanent abstention from enrichment, which the Iranian negotiators insisted could not be reported to their superiors as being under discussion.[43] For the sake of keeping the negotiations going, the E3 retained the evasive language and were willing to listen to Iranian proposals. It was the European view, however, strongly reinforced by Washington, that the only real objective guarantee would be the total cessation of the enrichment programme and any reprocessing activities. For both the Americans and Europeans, the logic was simple: if Iran cannot enrich uranium or reprocess plutonium, it cannot produce fissile material for a nuclear weapon. Any arrangement that allowed even limited enrichment would enable Iran to master the technologies and build a parallel clandestine facility and, further along the line, make weapons-grade uranium and withdraw from the NPT.

Iranian misinterpretation of European policy

Iranian diplomats and commentators contend that in late 2004, the Europeans had given up the goal of cessation and had conceded that Iran had a right to enrichment, before then being overruled by Washington in 2005 as a condition of US support for the E3 initiative.[44] This is a misreading. In fact, the quid pro quo for Washington's – sceptical – support was the E3's agreement to support immediate referral to the Security Council if Iran broke the 2004 suspension agreement. The Iranian view that the Europeans had been ready to accept enrichment appears to have been based at least in part on incomplete reporting by the Iranian negotiating team. Iran's chief negotiator and Secretary of the Supreme National Security Council Hassan Rowhani himself acknowledged in a May 2005 interview with an Iranian newspaper that the European goal from the beginning was an end to enrichment.[45]

Throughout the spring of 2005, the Iranians continued to misinterpret or misrepresent the European position, although perhaps with more justification than previously. In April, when Iran tabled a new proposal to resume uranium conversion and enrichment at a 3,000-centrifuge pilot plant and eventually to construct an industrial-scale enrichment plant of 50,000 centrifuges, in exchange for ratification of the Additional Protocol and acceptance of continuous on-site inspections at Natanz, the Europeans did not dismiss the proposal out of hand, so as not to rupture the negotiations. The Europeans were hoping to buy time until after the Iranian presidential elections of June 2005, which the pragmatic former President Hashemi Rafsanjani was expected to win. Thus they said that they were prepared to 'consider' Iran's proposal, but could not accept it as a basis for negotiations. European officials later remarked that the Iranians could not have been under any illusion that the proposal would have been acceptable.[46] French President Jacques Chirac was reported to have urged his negotiators to consider Iran's proposal that it be allowed to have an enrichment plant with 3,000 centrifuges,[47] but French officials insisted that France, the UK and Germany were 'rock solid on cessation' of Iran's uranium enrichment programme.[48] Various informal Iranian proposals that would allow Iran to complete the pilot-scale enrichment plant were consistently rejected.

Review proposals

Later in 2005, however, the Europeans did, at least in theory, move conclusively away from permanent cessation, and with American support. The E3 proposal for a long-term agreement made to Iran in August 2005, which included a long list of economic, political, nuclear-energy and other incentives, called on Tehran to make a 'binding commitment' not to pursue fuel-cycle activities other than nuclear reactors moderated by light water (which are less proliferation-sensitive than heavy-water reactors), but proposed that this commitment be reviewed every ten years.[49] However, Iran had by this time already resumed enrichment activity, and showed no interest in the proposal. A revised proposal submitted on 6 June 2006 by EU High Representative for the Common Foreign and Security Policy Javier Solana, now on behalf of the E3 plus China, Russia and the US, who had formally joined the negotiating group (making it the E3+3),[50] asked Iran to suspend its fuel-cycle activities during negotiations, and said that the long-term agreement to be negotiated, which would include a 'moratorium' (on enrichment), would be reviewed when 'international confidence in the exclusively peaceful nature of Iran's civil nuclear programme has been restored'.[51]

How it would be decided that confidence had been restored was not spelled out in the 2006 proposal. Iranians might have believed that nothing short of regime change would provide confidence enough for Washington hardliners. The Iranians were also surprised and suspicious about the change from a ten-year review cycle to the indefinite moratorium review mechanism of the 2006 proposal. When the incentives package was resubmitted to Iran in June 2008, the covering letter signed by the six foreign ministers and Solana suggested that continued lack of confidence was tied to the IAEA's inability 'to provide credible assurances about the absence of undeclared material and activities in Iran'. This could be read to mean that Iran's implementation of the Additional Protocol would be the basis for deciding whether confidence had been restored. The US, UK and France have maintained, however, that the judgement cannot be left up to the IAEA Secretariat alone.

The June 2008 offer also indicated that restoration of confidence would be a gradual process. Among the incentives offered was 'support for R&D in nuclear energy as international confidence is gradually restored'. Western officials privately acknowledge that this can be interpreted to mean that Iran may continue enrichment research and development while it suspends actual enrichment.[52]

Iran insists that it will not give up enrichment

Since talks on the issue began in 2003, Iran has never given any serious indication that it would be willing to give up the aim of acquiring enrichment technology, whatever inducements or disincentives the West might put forward. From 2003 to 2005, the government of President Mohammad Khatami was willing to suspend parts of the enrichment programme in exchange for the issue not being sent to the Security Council. Western nations hoped that this temporary suspension could be extended, little by little if need be, until months became years. Iranians feared just this – that prolonged suspension would become cessation by another name.[53] In summer 2005, after the E3 rejected a proposal for limits on centrifuge numbers with a phased expansion up to 50,000 machines and Mahmoud Ahmadinejad won a surprise victory over Rafsanjani in the presidential election, the outgoing Khatami government decided to end the suspension. Ever since, Iranian officials have insisted that suspension is non-negotiable because enrichment is the 'national will'. Having created this national will, the leadership insists it cannot now change it. Notwithstanding the circular logic of this position, there is no doubting the broad support in Iran for the enrichment goal. Former members of Khatami's government, as well as former President Rafsanjani and former chief negotiator Ali Larijani, have criticised Ahmadinejad's provocative statements and diplomatic ineptitude in handling the nuclear issue, but no prominent insiders are known to have criticised the programme itself or its ultimate aims.[54]

CHAPTER TWO

Western Strategy So Far

Denial of supply

For many years, the US-led strategy for impeding Iran's nuclear project was strictly supply-side, based on denying Iran the wherewithal to produce nuclear weapons. For nearly two decades, bilateral diplomacy to discourage potential suppliers coupled with multinational export controls effectively closed many of Iran's avenues to dual-use equipment of proliferation concern. Concerns about Iran's nuclear intentions grew in the 1990s, as evidence mounted about the country's interest in acquiring experimental uranium-isotope-separation equipment and heavy-water-moderated research reactors that appeared to be mainly intended to produce weapons-grade plutonium. Iran also sought to procure 'hot cell'-related equipment that would help its nuclear engineers learn how to process irradiated fuel to separate out the plutonium. There was even some evidence that Iran had sought to obtain fissile material or even nuclear weapons in the former Soviet Union.[1] But throughout the 1990s, the US was able to persuade Argentina, China, Kazakhstan and other countries not to sell Iran facilities or material that could be used for uranium enrichment or plutonium production.[2]

The US also used its leadership in the Nuclear Suppliers Group (NSG) to deny sensitive nuclear technology to Iran. Since the 1970s, the NSG has had an informal agreement not to sell enrichment or reprocessing technology to any developing country. In 1994, the NSG added to its formal guidelines a so-called 'non-proliferation principle' requiring suppliers to authorise a transfer only when satisfied that it would not contribute to proliferation. In 2004, the group added 'catch-all clauses' to the conditions of supply its members agreed to observe. Catch-all clauses prohibit the export of an item if the supplier has 'reason to believe' that it would be destined for a weapons purpose. These two rules commit member states to considering the proliferation credentials of recipient countries, thus furnishing a basis for singling out Iran. NSG members also conduct an active information exchange regarding Iranian procurement attempts and proliferation challenges. It is an indication of the NSG's effectiveness that between 1998 and 2007, seven of its members stopped a total of over 75 sales to Iran of dual-use nuclear-related materials.[3]

The denial strategy gained a higher public profile in May 2003 upon inauguration of the US-led Proliferation Security Initiative (PSI), which built on national maritime interdiction efforts and the ad-hoc multi-national cooperation that had been developing for several years to stop the illicit transfer of nuclear, chemical weapon- and missile-related goods. The PSI has helped to establish greater intelligence, diplomatic and operational coordination among its partner states, as well as among departments of government within states, and has reinforced states' capability to detain suspect cargo. How successful it has been in stopping any actual nuclear cargo bound for Iran is not easy to assess. In a May 2008 *Washington Times* op-ed, two former Bush administration senior officials responsible for the PSI said that 'dozens of interdictions have taken place slowing nuclear and missile programs in Asia and the Middle East'.[4] Typically, US declarations of successful PSI interdictions do not specify a country of destination, and it cannot be claimed that these interdictions would not have happened without the PSI. A May 2008 US briefing to a meeting marking the fifth anniversary of the PSI did give five detailed examples of PSI interdictions that had been claimed as successes. Only one of these – the denial by a European country of an export licence for coolers that could be used in Iran's heavy-water-reactor programme[5] – involved Iranian nuclear activity, and it was a diplomatic consultation of a kind that long predates the PSI. Notwithstanding the limited open-source accounting of successful interdictions, by strengthening individual and collective capabilities, PSI coordination has helped to strengthen the barriers to Iran's acquisition of dual-use goods. Tightening the interdiction regime to prevent Iranian import of dual-use technologies can directly help to restrict expansion of the enrichment programme.

Worst-case scenarios forestalled

As a result of these US-led denial efforts, dire predictions about the time-scale for Iran developing nuclear weapons have been repeatedly been proven wrong. Since the early 1990s, US intelligence agencies have been making what might be described as a rolling five-to-ten-year forecast of when Iran might acquire nuclear weapons. The fact that these worst-case scenarios did not come to pass does not represent an intelligence failure. Rather, it is a sign of intelligence success, as the predictions were based on assumptions about what Iran might be able to do if its efforts to acquire dual-use equipment were not thwarted.[6] And, with one major exception, they were thwarted. Intelligence estimates about when Iran could conceivably develop a nuclear weapon thus kept on being pushed back – until recently. A 2005 NIE concluded that 'early to mid-next decade' (i.e., 2010–15) was the earliest date by which Iran might be able to produce enough HEU for a weapon.[7] The November 2007 NIE moved the worst-case time frame forward, to the end of 2009.

Industrial sabotage

Industrial sabotage may have been another element of the denial strategy.[8] Taking advantage of Iran's reliance on black-market suppliers of components for its enrichment programme, Western intelligence agencies are said to have arranged for Iran to buy parts that were purposely designed with imperfections so that the centrifuges would not function properly. Two members of the Swiss family that played a key role in the Khan network, Urs and Marco Tinner, who have been under investigation and detained by Swiss investigative authorities for the past three years, reportedly told investigators that they were asked to manipulate parts for gas-centrifuge-pressure-regulation and UF_6-extraction systems as part of an undercover contract with the CIA.[9] The *New York Times* has reported that in 2003 and 2004, IAEA inspectors saw vacuum pumps in Iran that were 'damaged cleverly so that they looked perfectly fine but failed to operate properly' and that a sabotaged power supply from Turkey failed in early 2006, causing 50 centrifuges to explode.[10] In June 2008, an Iranian court gave a death sentence to Iranian businessman Ali Ashtari for what the court determined was espionage on behalf of Israel two years earlier, reportedly involving supplying 'defective and contaminated equipment' to the nuclear programme. According to an unnamed Iranian counter-intelligence official, 'in some instances the application of these parts led to the defeat of the project with irreversible damage'.[11] It has also been reported, but not confirmed, that the CIA and Mossad planned a joint operation to sabotage electricity supplies to Iranian nuclear sites[12] and that the CIA considered 'poisoning' computer networks used by the nuclear programme.[13]

Iran's evasion of controls via the black market
The exception to the successful effort to deny Iran foreign assistance with nuclear materials that might be used for weapons was, of course, its acquisition of Pakistani uranium-enrichment technology and equipment from the Khan black-market network. Though now well-known, it largely escaped the attention of Western intelligence at the time that Khan's global network was selling Iran cast-off Pakistani P-1 centrifuges from at least as early as 1987, later selling it plans and possibly models for P-2 machines. These clandestine sales enabled Iran to skip several stages of research-and-development work. Iran was also able to acquire components through other black-market suppliers that it continues to exploit. Today, with greater intelligence scrutiny, stricter export controls and UN sanctions, Iran is harder pressed to obtain goods on the black market. But no country is more active on the international black market than Iran. According to the Washington-based Institute for Science and International Security, 'Even today, the centrifuge program still acquires vacuum pumps and much of its measuring equipment via illicit trade with foreign suppliers.'[14]

Iran's ability to evade export controls by going through Khan and other illicit suppliers demonstrates the danger of a strategy focused exclusively on the supply side. By cracking down on illicit traffic and strictly regulating legitimate trade in sensitive items, concerned governments can alter the supply curve to the point where most black-market suppliers will have been driven out of the market. Evidence about recent Iranian procurements suggests that Iran is finding it harder to obtain the components it needs for its nuclear projects.[15] If the price is high enough, however, it is difficult to deny the economic adage that where there is a demand there is a supply. Success depends on many countries maintaining unwavering vigilance over exports. In a globalised economy, where not all states have the same degree of political commitment to export controls or the necessary customs detection and inspection capacity, Iran can exploit weak links in the chain.

Even illicit trade doors once thought closed to Iran may not have been so tightly shut. Evidence has emerged that, until recently, Russian entities may still have been transferring to Iran sensitive nuclear technology beyond that required for Bushehr. In a June 2008 statement to a congressional committee, former US Assistant Secretary of State for Nonproliferation Robert Einhorn remarked that:

Some such cooperation has reportedly taken place – and was the focus of high-level U.S. diplomatic efforts with Russian leaders … However, those diplomatic efforts, including during a March 2008 visit to Moscow by Secretary of State Condoleezza Rice and [Secretary of Defense] Robert Gates, have apparently resulted in strong assurances at the highest levels of the Russian government that any further sensitive cooperation between Russian entities and Iran will stop.[16]

Demand-side strategies

Positive inducements

To complement the supply-side denial tactics, European nations have led a strategy aimed at changing Iran's demand for sensitive nuclear technologies. Originally, this was focused on inducements, holding out the prospect of greater European trade and investment. Since 2001, negotiations on an EU–Iran Trade and Cooperation Agreement have been tied to changes to Iran's nuclear posture as well as to progress on human rights, terrorism and Iran's approach towards the Middle East peace process. The trade links between Iran and the West were strengthened in the November 2004 Paris Agreement. Also around this time, the Europeans began exploring other potential incentives for Iran to stop enrichment.

Meanwhile, from 2003, the US sought to add negative incentives to the demand-side strategy. Convinced that the European engagement approach was doomed to failure, the Bush administration stood apart from the process for four years, until 2005. The US instead pushed for Security Council sanctions from the moment in June 2003 when IAEA inspectors first documented Iran's failure to comply with its safeguards agreement. Some outside the US worried that the real objective of hard-line conservatives led by Vice President Dick Cheney was to work their way through UN sanctions options as quickly as possible in order to pave the way for their presumed preference of military action against Iran. The dominant Bush administration viewpoint, however, was that sanctioning Iran was the best way to persuade it change its policies. In 2005, the US accepted the European argument that sanctions needed to go hand-in-hand with inducements. Although this policy compromise was primarily a trade-off, made in return for the E3's agreement to bring Iran's case to the Security Council if inducements failed to halt enrichment activities, most US officials dealing with the issue accepted the need for both carrots and sticks.

In May 2006, the US agreed to a new package of incentives offered to Iran, this time by all six of the major powers. Presented in Tehran on 6 June by Javier Solana, the inducements included direct US engagement in the negotiations and offers of state-of-the-art nuclear technology, as well as refinements of the economic and political incentives that the E3 had – unsuccessfully – put forward in August 2005. Offering to join negotiations and, implicitly, to lift sanctions in any final accord with Iran was a major policy shift for the Bush administration, even if the promised benefits to Iran were not immediately tangible.

Iranian leaders did not find the offer of US engagement as enticing as the Europeans had expected. It may be that no American incentive would be sufficient to persuade Iran to give up its weapons option. In any case, Iran probably did not believe that Washington would in fact lift US sanctions or follow through with the other incentives. This would not have been an unreasonable assessment, given the antagonism towards Iran that prevails in the US Congress, which would have to approve any termination of sanctions. Iran also noted that the Americans had baulked at including in the 2006 offer the prospect of security assurances to Iran and guarantees of its territorial integrity, which the previous E3 offer had contained. Above all, the Iranians were unwilling to accept the precondition of a uranium-enrichment suspension, seeing it as a trap. They feared that Washington would pocket the suspension then make additional demands on missiles, terrorism, human rights, recognition of Israel and whatever else. The general perception in Tehran was that the proposals contained few guaranteed benefits for the Iranian side.[17]

Factors behind the 2003 halt in the weapons programme
The demand-side strategy is geared towards changing Iran's strategic analysis. In concluding that Iran had halted its nuclear-weaponisation programme in 2003, the November 2007 NIE judged that Iran's leaders were operating rationally, guided by a cost–benefit approach rather than an insistence on developing weapons at any cost, and that the decision to halt had been made in response to international scrutiny and pressure. This, the report said, suggests that some combination of threats and pressure, along with credible inducements, might prompt Iran to extend the halt, which the NIE judged 'with moderate confidence' had held at least up to mid 2007. The NIE also assessed, however, that convincing the Iranian leadership to forgo the eventual development of nuclear weapons altogether would be difficult.

The international scrutiny and pressure that Iran faced in 2003 was indeed intense and took several forms. In order to promote its goal of toppling the Islamic government, in August 2002, the Iranian exile group the National Council of Resistance of Iran had exposed (probably with Israeli help[18]) the secret nuclear facilities at Natanz, Esfahan and Arak. Subsequent IAEA investigations uncovered a string of safeguards violations and one inconsistency after another in Iran's explanations, giving the US ample grounds to push for UN sanctions. Iran at the same time faced newly triumphant US forces across one border in Iraq and another in Afghanistan. The doctrine of prevention that the US had enunciated in 2002, combined with the ease with which US-led forces had implemented that doctrine in overthrowing the Taliban the year before and Saddam Hussein in 2003, gave Tehran's leaders legitimate reason to fear that they would be targeted next. They would have seen the undisguised enthusiasm in US neo-conservative circles for moving on from Iraq to Iran, epitomised by sloganeering in the build-up to *Operation Iraqi Freedom* to the effect that 'real men go to Tehran'[19] and Under Secretary of State John Bolton's provocative message to Iran to 'take a number'.[20] The year 2003 saw the first congressional authorisation of funds – $1.5 million – to support NGOs inside Iran working for democracy and human rights. In late 2003, the Khan network was infiltrated, its October 2003 shipment to Libya was interdicted and its key associates were about to be arrested.[21] Although the end of the Khan network did not become public until February 2004, it is possible that Iran had reason in 2003 to suspect that the international dragnet was closing in on the network. Iran may also have known that Libyan leader Muammar Gadhafi was secretly negotiating with the UK and US to give up Libya's nuclear- and chemical-weapons programmes, a step that was announced on 19 December.

Sanctions and pressure

The US push for UN sanctions did not succeed until three and a half years after Iran's safeguards violations were first documented, and then only after a series of other diplomatic efforts reached a dead end. The timeline overleaf tracks events over this period.

The delay in adopting the first sanctions resolution reflected a European view that the threat of sanctions was more powerful than their actual imposition. Indeed, the sanctions threat had persuaded Iran to accept the first suspension agreement in October 2003 and the strengthened suspension agreement of November 2004. But once the issue was sent to the UN, Iran began to assign less value to the threat, realising that it could cope with the limited sanctions that the Security Council was able to muster.

Key dates relating to the Iranian nuclear issue, 2003–2006

- **6 June 2003:** IAEA reports Iran's failure to meet reporting obligations under its safeguards agreement.
- **19 June 2003:** IAEA Board calls on Iran not to start enrichment at Natanz.
- **12 September 2003:** First of six IAEA Board resolutions calling on Iran to suspend all enrichment-related activity, implicitly threatening referral to UN Security Council.
- **21 October 2003:** Tehran Agreement between the E3 and Iran, in which Iran agrees to suspend all enrichment and reprocessing activities as defined by the IAEA.
- **26 November 2003:** IAEA Board resolution defers a non-compliance finding.
- **29 December 2003:** Iran's definition of suspension makes clear that production and assembly of centrifuge machines is continuing.
- **23 February 2004:** E3–Iran Brussels Agreement, in which Iran agrees to extend scope of suspension.
- **13 March 2004:** IAEA Board resolution again defers non-compliance finding.
- **29 April 2004:** Iran begins 'hot test' of UF_6 production line at Esfahan.
- **18 May 2004:** After IAEA says hot test amounts to production of feed material for enrichment, Iran claims suspension does not include UF_6 production.
- **24 June 2004:** Iran resumes production and assembly of centrifuges.
- **16 August 2004:** Iran begins converting 37 tonnes of yellowcake into UF_6.
- **15 November 2004:** Paris Agreement between Iran and E3 – Iran agrees to comprehensive suspension of enrichment-related activities, including 'all tests or production at any uranium conversion facility'.[22]
- **29 November 2004:** IAEA Board resolution welcomes extension of suspension.
- **29 April 2005:** Iran threatens to resume uranium conversion.
- **25 May 2005:** Iran agrees to extend suspension pending presentation of E3 proposal in early August.
- **5 August 2005:** E3 proposes 31-page 'Framework for a Long-term Agreement', which includes a ten-year review mechanism for suspension.
- **8 August 2005:** Iran resumes uranium-conversion activity, abrogating the Paris Agreement.
- **24 September 2005:** IAEA Board finds Iran in non-compliance (by a vote of 22–1, with 12 abstentions); delays reporting to UN Security Council.
- **10 January 2006:** Iran resumes enrichment at Natanz.
- **4 February 2006:** IAEA Board votes to report Iran to the UN Security Council (by a vote of 27–3, with five abstentions).
- **5 February 2006:** Iran ceases implementation of the Additional Protocol and begins restricting inspector access to its sites.
- **29 March 2006:** UN Security Council issues statement calling on Iran to suspend all enrichment activities within a 30-day deadline.
- **6 June 2006:** Javier Solana presents E3+3 incentives package to Tehran.
- **4 July 2006:** Russian President Putin urges Iran to accept the E3+3 incentives package to ensure success of July G8 summit in St Petersburg. Iran responds with mixed signals.
- **31 July 2006:** Russia and China join in UN Security Council Resolution 1696 (adopted 14 –1), mandating under Chapter VII of UN Charter that Iran suspend enrichment activity, giving a 60-day deadline before further action is threatened.
- **28 September 2006:** Following Ayatollah Khamenei's rejection of chief negotiator Ali Larijani's proposal to offer a short suspension as a way of resuming formal negotiations, President Ahmadinejad states that Iran will not suspend uranium enrichment for 'a single day'.
- **23 December 2006:** UN Security Council Resolution 1737 applies first sanctions.

Russia and China consistently argued for milder sanctions than those pushed for by the UK, France and the US, and delayed their imposition. To begin with, Moscow and Beijing opposed the concept of sanctions altogether, viewing them as a tool that could too easily be used to infringe their own sovereignty. Both states seek to maintain friendly relations with Iran, primarily motivated in Russia's case by geostrategic considerations and in China's by its need for Iranian oil and gas. With the Iraq example fresh in their minds, Russia and China also saw sanctions and deadlines as a potential slippery slope to another destabilising war. Security Council sanctions, they felt, were often a one-way path to escalation, escalation which in this case could result in a push for military action by the West. Yet the Russians and Chinese do worry about the prospect of a nuclear-armed Iran, and so, however reluctantly, they joined the sanctions strategy. The political message this sent came as a psychological shock to Iran. Economically, however, sanctions have not had the intended impact. China bears responsibility for this in two ways. Along with Russia, China has prevented the adoption of measures that bite, and Chinese companies have stepped in to pick up some of the business opportunities spurned by Western firms. Anxious to avoid the lose–lose situation of losing national competitive advantage in addition to failing to impact on Iran's decision-making, many EU member states are highly reluctant to adopt unilateral sanctions measures.

Security Council sanctions resolutions

UNSCR 1737, passed unanimously on 23 December 2006, banned technical and financial assistance to Iran's enrichment, reprocessing, heavy-water and ballistic-missile programmes and froze the foreign-held assets of 12 Iranian individuals and ten Iranian organisations involved in those programmes. The resolution also put restrictions on IAEA technical cooperation with Iran and called on states to 'exercise vigilance' when allowing travel by Iranians involved in these activities and when dealing with Iranians seeking training in disciplines that would contribute to them.

UNSCR 1747 was passed with surprising speed on 24 March 2007, again with unanimity. It barred arms exports to Iran and doubled the number of Iranian entities subject to an asset freeze because of their involvement in Iran's nuclear and missile work, adding, among others, seven IRGC officers (in addition to one named in UNSCR 1737). Also on the list was Bank Sepah, Iran's fifth-largest bank, because of its transactions with Iranian entities named in UNSCR 1737. The individuals named in 1747 were not subject to a travel ban by the new resolution, but member states were obliged to report any entry to their territory of an individual sanctioned by the Council. It called on member states to 'exercise vigilance and restraint' in transferring arms to Iran. Most importantly, the resolution called on UN members not to enter into new commitments for grants or concessional loans to Iran. Although this was not mandatory, it provided a legal basis for states to apply financial pressure.

Enthused by the speed with which the second sanctions resolution had passed, the transatlantic allies hoped in summer 2007 that they could sustain the momentum of building pressure on Iran. But although Iran again ignored a deadline for suspension – this time the 60-day limit imposed by the latest resolution – a delay in sanctioning became inevitable when Ali Larijani resumed negotiations with Javier Solana and responded positively to efforts by the IAEA to work out a timetable for addressing its outstanding questions. Neither Russia nor China wanted another sanctions resolution tabled as long as Larijani was talking to Solana and working through the steps of the IAEA work plan. Release of the US NIE with its headline-grabbing assessment that Iran four years earlier had halted its single-purpose development work on nuclear weapons provided another reason to put off sanctions.

UNSCR 1803 was not adopted until 3 March 2008, after the US submitted to the IAEA additional documents detailing weaponisation studies and the IAEA reported that Iran, by refusing to answer questions about the alleged studies, had not allowed it to complete the work plan. Also, in January, Iran announced that it had begun work on advanced centrifuge designs. Concerns about the weaponisation work and the new-generation centrifuges provided a political basis for the third sanctions resolution, which passed 14–0 (Indonesia abstaining). This resolution added 13 names to the previous list of 17 Iranian entities subject to an asset freeze and travel ban, and prohibited trade with Iran in certain dual-use materials and technologies. It also authorised the inspection of shipments suspected of containing banned items carried by an Iranian airline and a shipping company, and called for vigilant monitoring of the activities of certain Iranian financial institutions.

UNSCR 1835, adopted unanimously on 27 September 2008, repeated the previous demands to suspend enrichment and reprocessing and to cooperate with the IAEA, but added no new sanctions or any new deadline. Intended to demonstrate that the Council remained unified, the resolution was quickly adopted once Russia had made clear that it would not accept anything harsher. By this time, the list of cost-free potential sanctions had largely been exhausted. Reaching agreement on new sanctions that would impose costs on the sanctioning as well as the sanctioned parties would have been very difficult even before Russia's relations with the West deteriorated in the aftermath of the Georgia crisis. Western leaders were thankful for almost any resolution.

EU and other non-UN sanctions
Following each of the sanctions resolutions, the EU adopted its own set of stronger measures extending the UN sanctions. In 2007, the EU followed up on UNSCRs 1737 and 1747 by freezing the assets of 20 additional entities and individuals not on the UN list and enacting a more comprehensive arms embargo on Iran and a travel ban on more Iranian officials than had been required by the UN. In further follow-up to UNSCR 1747 in June 2008, the EU froze the assets of Bank Melli, Iran's largest bank, as well as 12 other entities. In August, the EU went slightly beyond the provisions of UNSCR 1803 by calling on its member states to 'exercise restraint in entering into new commitments for public-provided financial support for trade with Iran', and to 'exercise vigilance over the activities of financial institutions within their jurisdiction with banks domiciled in Iran'.[23] Also in August, in response to UNSCR 1803, the EU authorised member states to step up checks on Iran-bound ships and aircraft in cases where there was suspicion that they were carrying banned goods. In October, Australia too decided to go beyond the UN sanctions, banning transactions with 20 Iranian officials and 18 Iranian entities, including Bank Melli and Bank Saderat.[24]

US financial pressure
Separate from the Security Council sanctions route, the US has engaged in a determined campaign to impose costs on Iran by limiting its access to the international business sector. This campaign of financial isolation involves both legal action taken to officially bar Iranian entities from the US financial system and informal pressure on foreign firms not to conduct business with Iran.

The campaign began in earnest in June 2005, when the US government adopted a legal instrument, Executive Order 13382, to enable the president to authorise the secretary of state and the Treasury secretary to freeze the assets of any foreign persons deemed to have engaged in or supported the proliferation of weapons of mass destruction, and to deny them any transactions with US entities. Three Iranian entities, including the Atomic

Energy Organisation of Iran, were on the initial list of 28 June 2005. A dozen more were designated in 2006 and 2007, including Bank Sepah (in January 2007) and Bank Melli, Bank Mellat, the IRGC, the Ministry of Defence and the Armed Forces Logistics and the Defence Industries Organisation (all designated on October 2007). Eleven more Iranian names were added on 8 July 2008, followed by five on 12 August, 19 on 10 September (the Islamic Republic of Iran Shipping Lines plus 18 affiliates) and four on 22 October (the Export Development Bank of Iran and three associated institutions), bringing the total to 69.[25] A separate authority, Executive Order 13224, was used in October 2007 to deny Bank Saderat and the IRGC–Qods Force (an elite military unit established for foreign operations) access to US financial systems on the grounds of their support for terrorism. None of these entities was known to have had any assets in the US subject to seizure. By taking this action, however, the US hoped to blackball the named companies and to persuade other governments to take similar action.

The most effective steps have been US Treasury efforts to directly affect private-sector investment decisions through pressure and suasion. When the US Treasury fined Dutch bank ABN Amro $80m in December 2005 for failing to fully report the processing of financial transactions involving Bank Melli in compliance with US sanctions legislation, it sent a clear warning to others. Efforts to persuade international companies of the wisdom of keeping Iran at arm's length have been backed up by formal cautions issued by the US Financial Crimes Enforcement Network and the international Financial Action Task Force (FATF), aimed at convincing firms that Iran is not a good place to do business. FATF advisories in October 2007 and February 2008 called on all of the organisation's member states to advise their financial institutions about the risks posed by deficiencies in Iran's anti-money-laundering and anti-terrorism-financing regimes.[26] According to the US Treasury, the UK, Canada, France, Germany, Japan and Malaysia are among the countries that have advised their financial institutions of the risks associated with doing business with Iran.[27]

As a result of this pressure, by the end of 2007, Japan's three largest banks, Switzerland's two largest banks, Germany's three largest banks and the UK's largest and sixth-largest banks had either ceased operations in Iran or stopped taking on new business in the country. France's BNP Paribas and Calyon, the investment-banking arm of Crédit Agricole, stopped offering letters of credit on Iranian fuel imports in 2007,[28] and in summer 2008 Natexis, one of France's largest banks, announced that it was pulling out of Iran completely. Overall, French banks reduced their exposure to Iran from $5.8bn in March 2006 to $1.9bn in mid 2007.[29] Most of

Kuwait's banks have reportedly stopped dealing with Iranian accounts.[30] The number of foreign banks operating in Iran has sharply declined since 2006, dropping from 46 to 20.[31] Chinese banks are among those that have reduced their commitments.

Business withdrawal

Many European industrial groups, including British Petroleum, ABN Amro and Siemens, have stopped new investments in and dollar transactions with Iran. In October 2006, Japan's INPEX Holdings pulled out of a deal to develop the Azadegan oilfield in Iran. In May 2008, Royal Dutch Shell and the Spanish oil company Repsol pulled back from investing in the development of the South Pars natural gas field, one of Iran's biggest gas projects.[32] In July 2008, the French energy giant Total abandoned talks on developing a liquefied natural gas project in Iran.[33] In each of these cases, companies made a business decision that continuing with their existing investment strategies was too risky in light of US pressure, UN sanctions and EU guidelines.

Not all European companies have stopped business with Iran, however. In April 2007, Austrian energy company OMV closed a €22bn deal with Iran for investment in South Pars in exchange for liquefied natural gas. In March 2008, Swiss energy company EGL signed a contract with Iran for gas supply worth up to €27bn. At least 1,700 German firms were still active in Iran in 2007, selling more than $5bn-worth of goods, and the German Office for Foreign Trade was still promoting trade opportunities for the capital goods that Iran was eager to buy.[34] In July 2008, German energy company SPG Steiner Prematechnik Gastec signed a €100m deal to build three plants for liquefied natural gas production, after the German government ruled that the agreement did not violate sanctions.[35] Russia's Gazprom continues to explore an energy deal with Iran, reportedly hoping to take advantage of European firms pulling out.[36] Companies from Malaysia, China, Turkey and India have made preliminary deals to expand Iran's energy-export prospects, although not all of these have been implemented.[37]

Other sanctions under consideration

Additional measures being considered, particularly by the US, France and the UK, include:

- *Adding more Iranian banks to the list of banned entities.* The two banks most vulnerable to a freeze of assets by European governments are Bank Mellat, designated for sanctioning by the US Treasury in

October 2007 for providing banking services to Iran's nuclear entities, and Bank Saderat, over whose activities UNSCR 1803 called upon states to exercise vigilance. The Central Bank of Iran has also been considered for sanctions by US and European governments, on the grounds that it provides financial services to banned banks, encourages them to conceal their involvement in nuclear and missile programmes[38] and has taken over some of the questionable business they have had to shed. However, US Treasury Deputy Assistant Secretary Daniel Glaser testified in Congress in April 2008 that while sanctioning the central bank was an option, it was an extraordinary step that the US was not yet ready to take.[39]

- *Extending financial pressure to other parts of the Iranian economy.* The financial isolation strategy that has so far been primarily directed at Iran's banking industry could be expanded to include its insurance, shipping, freight-forwarding and import–export sectors. The US, UK and France are considering a plan to persuade international insurance companies to withdraw coverage from Iranian cargo shipments, infrastructure and businesses rather than face the 'reputational risks' of maintaining links with Iran.[40] The reinsurance subsector, which insures the insurers, is likely to be a particular target of any such plan, because the small number of companies in the business are concentrated in the US, UK and France. Whichever sectors are targeted, regulators in Western countries will try to persuade companies that, because of the deceptive practices used in the past by Iranian banks to avoid detection of proliferation-related financing and the degree to which the IRGC uses front companies to conduct its international business, they cannot be certain that business conducted with any Iranian company does not have a connection to proliferation or terrorism.

- *Strictly implementing existing measures.* In its August 2008 statement on financial dealings with Iran, the EU called for member states to exercise vigilance over the transactions with Iranian banks undertaken by financial institutions in their jurisdiction. As the US has already taken such a step with its own banks, strict implementation of this measure by European governments would deny Iran access to the world's largest financial centres. Implementation is more likely to the degree that states believe it will have an impact on Iran and forestall Israeli or US military action.

- *Banning EU investment in selected sectors.* In November 2007, UK Prime Minister Gordon Brown called for sanctions on investment in Iran's dominant revenue earner, the oil and gas industry,[41] which is already suffering from declining production because of a lack of enhanced oil-recovery techniques. Rather than a global ban on all such investment, which China and Russia would not support, discussions have focused on an EU and US ban on investment in the petroleum-refining and liquefied petroleum gas industries, in which Western firms have the leading technology. Opposition from Germany, in particular, has prevented adoption of this measure to date, but it is still under discussion. Sanctions that hamper Iran's ability to produce gas and oil are not cost-free, given the global demand for increased oil supply.

- *Embargoing refined petroleum imports.* Stopping the petrol imports that fuel 40% of Iran's road transport could, in theory, be the most effective way of influencing the country's cost–benefit calculations. The resulting rise in petrol prices would immediately drive home to ordinary citizens the high cost of the nuclear policy. It has been reported that US pressure has already prompted India's largest private petroleum refiner to stop supplying Iran.[42] Yet an embargo would pose daunting implementation challenges. Because Iran's petrol suppliers are so diverse – coming from Gulf countries, India, Turkey, Central Asia, Europe, Russia, China and Venezuela – and the product is fungible, a ban on refined oil sales would be inherently leaky.

- *Divesting from companies doing business with Iran.* In the US, a campaign led by Israel-affiliated lobby groups seeks to force the $1 trillion pension-fund industry to divest from multilateral companies with business in Iran. In particular, the divestment advocates hope to deprive Tehran of investment in its declining oil and gas infrastructure. By July 2008, 11 US states had adopted divestment legislation and another 20 were considering similar bills.[43] California's law divested as much as $24bn in pension-fund assets from energy and defence companies doing business with Iran. (The law was limited to those sectors.) In 2008, Congress was considering legislation that would give legal protection to money managers undertaking such divestments.

- *Banning export credits.* Over the past few years, the US has repeatedly urged the EU to put an end to the government-backed insurance credits that underpin a significant amount of business with Iran. While the UK and France support such a ban, several other European states have consistently resisted adopting a formal ban. Most of them have, however, sharply reduced new export credits. From 2008, the UK ceased processing applications for new export-credit cover to Iran.[44] Italy quietly stopped issuing new insurance credits in 2007.[45] Germany, which issued about $2bn in export credits for trade with Iran in 2005, reduced new credits to around $715m in 2007.[46] In late 2007, Germany's total credit commitment, designed to assist small and medium-sized companies, was still around €5bn, while the UK's exposure was around a tenth of that amount.[47]

- *Intensifying financial pressure on IRGC branches.* Those European states that have applicable anti-terrorism legislation, such as the UK's Terrorism Act of 2000, have been encouraged to take action similar to America's in subjecting the IRGC-Qods Force to a financial ban.[48] It has also been suggested that sanctions be imposed on Iranian companies controlled by the IRGC, for example the huge engineering firm Khatam ol-Anbia, which has a $2bn contract to develop parts of the South Pars natural gas field and a $1.3bn contract to build parts of a pipeline.[49]

- *Banning all arms sales.* More than almost any other measure, an embargo on the conventional arms on which the Iranian military depends would give the leadership a reason to rethink the nuclear strategy. Western attempts to impose a complete arms-trade ban on Iran have been blocked by Russia, Iran's chief weapons supplier. Since 2001, Russia has signed over $1bn of new arms agreements with Iran.[50]

There is no shortage of pundit recommendations for other pressure tactics, many of which Western states could adopt without Russian and Chinese support. These include restricting air travel to and from Iran, requiring strict inspection of all Iranian ships and aircraft to prevent sanctions violations, withdrawing support for Iran's membership of the World Trade Organisation (WTO), disqualifying Iranian teams from international competitions,[51] withholding spare parts for European-supplied factory equipment[52] and suspending the sale of spare parts for the European cars that dominate Iranian roads.[53] Former US Middle East envoy Dennis Ross advocates enlisting Saudi Arabia by encouraging it to use its financial and petrochemical leverage to persuade its trading partners, including Russia, China and the United Arab Emirates (UAE), to cut back on trade with Iran.[54]

US and Israeli military pressure

The US and Israel have also sought to influence Iran's cost–benefit calculations by raising the spectre of military action. For example, US naval exercises in the Gulf in March 2007 by two carrier strike groups were part of a regular training schedule, but they also served to remind Iran of the US naval power that is available if called upon, notwithstanding the degree to which US ground forces are overstretched by duty in Iraq and Afghanistan.

In summer 2007, US Vice President Dick Cheney's office was widely rumoured to be intent on using confrontation with Iranian operatives in Iraq as an excuse for 'hot pursuit' into Iran and using the further escalation that would follow to reach the stage of attacking Iran's nuclear installations. Whether or not there was any truth in these rumours, they served as a 'psychological operation' to further remind Iran of the potential for US military action, including both air strikes and a naval embargo. Israel's September 2007 bombing of the Syrian nuclear reactor at al-Kibar served a similar purpose of demonstrating to Iran that Israel had both the will and the capability to destroy nuclear facilities that posed a potential proliferation threat. Although the release of the November 2007 NIE put to rest the prospect of US-led military action against Iran, by mid 2008, Israeli sabre-rattling was stimulating renewed talk of the possibility of air strikes. An Israeli military exercise in the Mediterranean in June 2008, in which 100 jets rehearsed the bombing of a distant target and helicopters simulated the rescue of downed pilots, sent an unmistakable signal to Iran that could not be entirely dismissed as propaganda. The factors influencing Israeli thinking about the timing of any attack were said to include not only Iran's advancing mastery of the enrichment process, but also the schedule for delivery to Iran of new Russian-made SA-20 anti-aircraft missiles, the projected early-2009 start-up date for the Bushehr reactor (after which bombing it could create an environmental catastrophe), and the political window of opportunity that was felt to be presented by the interregnum between the US presidential election in early November and the late January inauguration of the new president. Israel's hints about its preparedness to attack were not only directed at Iran, but also – and perhaps even more so – at the rest of the world, as a warning to other nations that if they did not take serious action to stop Iran's enrichment activities, Israel would be forced to rely on its own means.

Iranians typically react to such psychological warfare with public nonchalance. In early July 2008, Ahmadinejad called talk of war a 'funny joke'.[55] Other statements by senior leaders, however, indicate that Iran does not totally dismiss the danger. At around the same time as Ahmadinejad made his remark, current Chairman of the Expediency Council Hashemi Rafsanjani told state-run Iranian television that 'Iran cannot ignore threats as mere psychological warfare'.[56] Iran responded to Israel's June 2008 exercise with its own show of steel. In early July, it undertook multiple missile tests to show that it had ample retaliatory options, although the public display backfired when one of the missiles failed to launch and was digitally added to a photograph of the test launches released by the IRGC news website.

Is the strategy working?

However much Iran's nuclear programme was impeded in the past, Western strategies have failed in the past five years to prevent Iran from acquiring a uranium-enrichment capability. European negotiators persuaded Iran to stop (some) enrichment-related work for intermittent periods between 2003 and 2005, and sanctions and export controls have prevented Iran from procuring all the items it has been seeking for its nuclear and missile programmes. Iran has also been persuaded to change its approach to cooperation with the IAEA, a change exemplified by the work plan of August 2007. But it has not deviated from its enrichment goal. MIT-based nuclear non-proliferation expert Jim Walsh is among those who argue that 'there is overwhelming evidence that the policy is not working. Moreover, the policy is unlikely to work within a timeframe that is relevant to the nuclear issue'.[57] He and former US Ambassadors William Luers and Thomas Pickering contend that the 'strategy of containment and sanctions, while irritating to the Iranian regime, will prove irrelevant to the country's nuclear programs', and that 'every centrifuge that Iran builds – whether it works or not – creates new facts on the ground'.[58]

In 2007, Iran rapidly expanded its centrifuge programme, going from around 250 machines in November 2006 to nearly 3,000 a year later. In 2008, it rapidly improved the operation of its centrifuge cascades, moving from 20% to 85% of claimed capacity (based on the UF_6 feed rate).[59] By 7 November, Iran had produced 630kg of LEU, and was adding more than 2kg a day to this total.[60] Under optimal conditions, around 700kg–800kg of LEU is needed to make the approximately 20kg of 93% HEU required for a nuclear weapon.[61] This means that, theoretically at least, Iran could possess the necessary quantities within a few months.

The West's failure thus far to stop Iran does not mean that Iran is 'winning'. Although many Iranians would claim that successful defiance of the West is victory enough, defiance comes at the high cost of political and economic isolation. The outcome so far can best be characterised as 'lose–lose'. For the rest of the world, the costs include a loss of transparency in Iran's nuclear programme, with Tehran responding to sanctions with sharply reduced cooperation with the IAEA. Overall, the US and its British and French allies contend that it is too early to conclude that Western policy has failed, because it has not yet been fully implemented, especially as regards the more biting sanctions.

Tactical successes for the West

The West can point to some tactical successes. Foremost among these is the maintenance of transatlantic unity, and consensus among the five permanent members of the UN Security Council. Indeed, the near unanimity of Security Council resolutions – with only one 'no' vote and one abstention in the five resolutions on Iran tabled up to 2008 – and the decisive votes of the IAEA Board of Governors appear to indicate that the broader international community has concluded that Iran's nuclear programme presents a problem. Iranian officials contest this, claiming that most countries in fact side with Iran. They cite as recent proof of this the declaration of a ministerial conference of the 118-member Non-Aligned Movement (NAM), held in Tehran 30 July 2008, which states that Iran's 'fuel cycle policies must be respected'.[62] The NAM statement was watered down from the version Iran originally sought, however, a process that included the excision of a description of UN sanctions on Iran as 'political'.[63]

Internal debate in Iran

In terms of the psychological impact within Iran, the unanimity of the first two sanctions resolutions (and the near unanimity of the third) was more important than their actual content. There is very little public dissent about the goal and substance of the nuclear programme – challenging the enrichment programme in print is forbidden – but Security Council action did at least succeed in initiating a debate within Iran. Challenges to the government's handling of the nuclear portfolio have flared episodically in public discourse. The first wave of open criticism came in the immediate aftermath of the passage in December 2006 of the first UN Security Council sanctions resolution, which provoked more dismay in Iran than Western policymakers had expected. The decision of its erstwhile protectors, Russia and China, to line up with the West in imposing sanctions shocked Iran. A newspaper connected with Supreme Leader Khamenei accused Ahmadinejad of endangering public support for the nuclear programme by hijacking it as a personal cause and criticised him for being dismissive of the sanctions resolution, which it said was 'certainly harmful to our country'.[64] The parliament, known as the Majlis, held a public debate on whether the defiant attitude of the government was furnishing a basis for additional sanctions. Treading into dangerous territory, a major reformist party, the Islamic Participation Front, called for a public discussion to inform the people of the depth and scope of the costs and benefits of the nuclear programme, while former nuclear negotiator Hossein Mousavian warned that Iran could not ignore the Security Council. In response, the government cracked down, jailing Mousavian for espionage (of which he was later acquitted) and silencing critics by stirring up fears of conflict with the US.

Criticism of Ahmadinejad's handling of the nuclear issue re-emerged in late October 2007, after the president replaced Ali Larijani as chief nuclear negotiator with his confidant and deputy foreign minister, the ineffectual Saeed Jalili. A letter criticising the appointment was signed by 183 members of the Majlis. Former chief negotiator Hassan Rowhani, who remains a member of the Supreme National Security Council, delivered an unusually sharp rebuke, saying that the president's policies were turning more countries against Iran and failing to fix the struggling economy. Speaking to the pro-reform Moderation and Development Party, Rowhani did not directly mention Ahmadinejad, but was clearly referring to his policies: 'On the international stage, we are under threat more than any other time ... Unfortunately, the number of our enemies are increasing.'[65] In a December newspaper interview he went further: 'We cannot open a letter of credit, is this power? An Iranian student cannot study abroad in a chosen field, is this power? The fact that the economic risks have grown, is that power? The fact that banking activities have been restricted, is this power?'[66] In response, Ahmadinejad denounced as traitors those countrymen who criticised the nuclear programme.

In casting Western demands on the nuclear project as an affront to Iranian pride, Iran's leaders have bet successfully on nationalism trumping economics. According to one line of thinking, Iranian hardliners are strengthened by US pressure, because it provokes a nationalistic response and makes enemies of the Iranian people.[67] Jim Walsh argues that 'sanctions give Iranian leaders a scapegoat for their own economic mismanagement'.[68] The threat of military attack in particular may offer a strong impetus to band together, bridging internal disagreements and contradictions.[69] There is evidence, however, that the domestic debate is continuing. Following the passage of UNSCR 1803, Majlis member and director of the Strategic Majlis Research Centre, Ahmad Tavakkoli, criticised the government's foreign policy, saying that 'the recent sanctions cost us a great deal' and that 'moderate conduct and rational and wise negotiations within the framework of foreign policies can reduce the costs for us'.[70]

The debate became more intense after 16 June 2008, when the E3+3 presented a repackaged version of its June 2006 incentives, along with a renewed proposal for a so-called 'double freeze' – no additional sanctions and no additional centrifuges (first proposed in summer 2007) – as a basis for a six-week period of 'pre-negotiations', to be followed by a full suspension during full negotiations. Former Foreign Minister Ali Velayati, a top adviser to the Supreme Leader, issued a warning against making any provocative statements, and declared that Iran should accept the package. Iranian state radio held an unprecedented debate on whether or not to do so. Describing such responses, US Under Secretary of State for Political Affairs William Burns told a congressional committee in July 2008 that 'it's hard to say where any of this will lead, but it at least suggests that it is well worth the effort to explain and publicize what we are putting on the table.'[71]

The economic impact of sanctions

Iran is in significant economic difficulty: unemployment is high (officially counted at 10.3% in March 2007,[72] but considered by some knowledgeable observers to be as high as 15%[73]) and inflation had risen to nearly 30% by September 2008. In 2007, the OECD revised Iran's credit risk rating from five to six on a scale of nought to seven, as a result of which the cost of export credits to Iran increased by 30%, and the overall level of credit diminished.[74] In September 2006, Oil Minister Kazem Vaziri-Hamaneh suggested that without new investment – which has not been forthcoming – output from Iran's oilfields would fall by around 13% a year.[75]

While Iranian leaders now accept that sanctions play a role in the country's economic trouble, just how much of the problem can be attributed to sanctions is difficult to measure. Ahmadinejad's mismanagement of the economy, notably through subsidies that fuel inflation and favouritism to state companies that drives out private enterprise, bears much of the responsibility for Iran's economic malaise. Conversely, the high price of oil that prevailed until autumn 2008 had a greater impact on the Iranian economy than did sanctions and Iran's role as a leading oil and gas exporter shielded it from much economic pressure.[76] Now, if oil prices stay below $95 a barrel, the resulting budget deficit[77] will exacerbate the impact of Western financial pressure. In any case, there is no doubt that Western pressure has been hurting. Even before the UN sanctions were imposed, an Iranian parliamentary report of September 2006 warned about the destabilising impact of sanctions, which it estimated were costing the Iranian economy $1.5–$2bn a year.[78] Over the four months to February 2008, commodity prices reportedly rose by 50% as a result of the extra cost of routing business through Dubai.[79] Iran's business community cannot get letters of credit or set up bank-transfer arrangements for international transactions, and must use cash rather than electronic transfers. Barter arrangements are becoming normal. Instead of lobbying for the government to change the policies that provoke the sanctions, however, businessmen are asking for compensation in the form of lower taxes, free transport of goods and the lifting of customs duties.

Iran has been able to anticipate the incremental sanctions that have been imposed on it and to find ways of eluding many of them. Discouraged members of the more moderate administration of previous president Mohammad Khatami have lamented privately that the hardliners were proven right – 'that Iran could get away with continued enrichment without the sky falling in'.[80] Shortly before the EU freeze on the assets of Bank Melli was imposed, Iran reportedly moved $75bn out of European banks.[81] To replace its reliance on European financial institutions, Iran has increasingly turned to smaller, second-tier banks in Dubai and Bahrain – and further afield in China, Southeast Asia and Latin America – that place less emphasis on reputational risk. After the Security Council passed its third set of sanctions in March 2008, Iranian Economy Minister Davoud Danesh-Jafari remarked that 'if we had any special difficulty in opening credit for merchants, the volume of investment in the country would not have increased compared with last year'.[82] But the US has been successful in twisting the arms of several banks in developing countries. In early 2008 it was reported that Bahrain's largest lender, Ahli United Bank, had frozen banking activity with Iran, and that lenders in the UAE had been holding off on issuing letters of credit to Iranian companies.[83]

The time factor

Timescales are critical to the Iran policy debate. The policy goal for the West is to stop the enrichment programme before it can produce nuclear weapons, or at least to slow it down enough that this day remains in the future. But what does this mean in practice, and how would the rest of the world know when Iran had reached that red line? If and when it happens, will Western policy have been overtaken by events and rendered obsolete?

Iran's enrichment programme has already reached the stage that in Israeli policy circles used to be called the 'point of no return'. When it was popularised in the early part of the decade, this term denoted the point at which Iran had mastered the enrichment process and had sufficient materials on hand to be able to enrich significant quantities of uranium without foreign assistance. At that point, Iran would be able either to produce HEU in clandestine facilities or to build up stockpiles of LEU in declared facilities that could be further enriched to HEU if it broke out of the NPT. Self-sufficiency would make the programme immune from sanctions and embargoes. Once such a point as this has been reached, achieving a weapons capability is only a matter of time and the politics of deciding to cross the threshold. But the 'no return' term is a misnomer in more ways than one. Talking about a point of no return incorrectly implies that states never turn back from nuclear-weapons mastery. It is true that knowledge once acquired cannot be 'unlearned' (without assassination of an entire scientific community). But states can and have decided to cease applying such knowledge, as in South Africa in 1990. Moreover, there is no single point at which enrichment can be said to be 'mastered'; it is a matter of learning curves, not breakthrough moments. The phrase thus posits a false deadline. Recognising these problems, Israeli policymakers and analysts stopped using the term in 2006, replacing it with 'techno-logical threshold'.[84] The concept, however, is the same, as is the purpose of emphasising it: to influence the diplomatic process by urging the West that time is short and must be used wisely.[85] Both terms are fuzzy and elastic, and have sometimes been overstated for effect, with inevitable drawbacks. It is counterproductive to emphasise a red line that is either on the verge of being crossed or has already been crossed, as this removes the utility of the term as a public-diplomacy tool. The red line most frequently cited by commentators today is the point at which Iran can make enough HEU to build a bomb, before which it is often said that action must be taken – by Israel alone if need be.[86] As noted above, depending on how much enriched uranium is needed, that day may come within a matter of months.

Iran is well along its learning curve, though how far along is a matter of perspective and debate. The country's leaders frequently make exagger-ated claims about the achievements of the enrichment programme. Western government officials typically downplay Iran's progress, pointing up the technical difficulties that Iran continues to face. The rush to install centrifuges in the main enrichment facility at Natanz while it was still under construction, rather than in the clean-room environment that delicate machines of this type need, gave Western officials reason to conclude that Iran's haste was making for waste. The sort of analysis that emphasises such shortcomings has seemed at times to be infused with hope. By belittling Iran's claims, Western officials could convince themselves that there was still time for their strategies to work. To say that there is still time is also to acknowledge, however, that the day may come when time has run out.

The operation of one 'unit' of 3,000 centrifuges – the stage reached by Iran in late 2007 – is commonly seen as marking the cut-off point between pilot-plant operation and industrial-scale enrichment. This rule of thumb does not mean that 3,000 machines are either necessary or sufficient for weapons production. The production of enough HEU for a chain reaction is made possible by a combination of numbers, efficiency and time; altering one of these factors can compensate for limitations in the others. The effectiveness of the centrifuge (measured in separative work units, SWUs) can be more important than the number of machines. Capabilities are assessed not by the number of machines available but by the quantity of SWUs that can be produced. In the case of ultra-modern American research-and-development centrifuges, which are 150 times as efficient as the P-1 model used by Iran, as few as three machines can produce enough HEU for a weapon, using batch processing.[87]

If the enrichment programme were for commercial purposes, Iran should have operated the cascades continuously for much longer periods of time and improved their efficiency before beginning the industrial-scale production that it started in 2007. It can be years before it is clear whether an enrichment programme is working well – Japan's centrifuge machines at the Rokkasho-mura plant started to crash seven years after installation.[88] If Iran's purpose is to quickly stockpile enough LEU for a military breakout, however, the long-term viability of the machines is less relevant.

Unknown centrifuge-production capability
On 8 April 2008, designated as National Nuclear Day, Ahmadinejad announced that Iran had started to install another 6,000 centrifuges at Natanz. The IAEA reported in May that installation work was under way on these 6,000 plus two other units of 3,000, which would make a total of 15,000 centrifuges (including those already in place).[89] Eventually, Natanz is planned to hold 54,000 machines.[90] Equipping such an industrial-scale

plant would probably take Iran a decade, even if it could produce that many centrifuges. A plant of this size would give Iran a quick break-out capability – that is, the ability to produce, on withdrawal from the NPT, a few bombs' worth of HEU in anything between a few weeks and as little as two or three days, depending on whether it was starting from natural, unenriched uranium or LEU.[91] Whether Iran can indigenously produce several thousand more centrifuges is thus a key intelligence question with important policy implications.

The E3+3 'double freeze' proposal was premised on the belief that it is important at least to stop the number of cascades from increasing. Iran did not accept the proposal (which is formally still on the table), even after signalling in June 2008 that it would – a signal that led the US to send Under Secretary of State William Burns to Geneva on 19 July with the other E3+3 partners for pre-talks with Iran's chief nuclear negotiator that went nowhere. Iran would appear to have little to lose from accepting the capping proposal, because existing machines would continue to operate, allowing Iranian engineers to continue progress towards mastering the enrichment process. Though it was cast as strictly a temporary measure, the double-freeze proposal, were it to be accepted, could conceivably carry on for longer, and become a de-facto redefinition of suspension. If there is no bottleneck obstructing Iran's centrifuge-production capability, then capping centrifuge numbers as a way of strengthening the barrier to break-out is a worthy policy objective. If Iran is unable to produce certain components, however, then the size of the programme will be limited in any case by the extent to which it can procure such components on the black market. In this situation, any deal to simply cap the programme would be a bargain of little value.

A good estimate of the number of centrifuges that Iran could make is important for assessing the likely effectiveness of any air strikes. If Iran had the capacity to make many more centrifuges than the quantity now installed, an air strike that destroyed the Natanz facility would not cripple its enrichment programme for very long. An August 2008 report of the Institute for Science and International Security assessed that:

> Iran has ... had ample time to accumulate large stocks of complete centrifuges and related equipment and materials. If they are not already in storage at interim locations or in underground or protected sites, they could be moved to such sites relatively quickly. ... Iran's manufacturing complex is able to replicate centrifuges relatively quickly and in large numbers.[92]

In 2005, when the IAEA still had access to Iran's centrifuge-manufacturing workshops, it conducted an inventory of centrifuge parts that, according to senior agency diplomats in Vienna, were together enough to make 10,000 machines, although many of these would have been of poor quality.[93] Since then, Iran has been able to produce many more parts. Having been denied access to components and centrifuge workshops since February 2006, the IAEA cannot confirm Iran's claims that it is able to manufacture all the nearly 100 components required for each centrifuge. The head of an Iranian company working on advanced P-2 centrifuges told the IAEA in 2004 that all the components for that model were produced domestically except for bearings, special oils and magnets.[94] Whether this is still the case, and whether the same limits on domestic production apply to the P-1 or the IR-2 and IR-3 centrifuge models also used, is unclear. Western intelligence agencies apparently do not know. An inability to produce all speciality components on its own would not be an obstacle if Iran were able to procure sufficient quantities from the black market. Although Iran probably cannot produce the high-strength maraging steel needed for the bellows for its P-1 and IR-3 centrifuges, for example, it possesses 67 tonnes illicitly acquired from the UK in the 1990s, enough for more than 30,000 centrifuges.[95] Looking at all the data, the Institute for Science and International Security researchers assess that Iran could probably produce up to 10,000 P-1 centrifuges with the materials it has on hand, and might be able to produce more than this number.[96]

The red line of LEU accumulation
Although the November NIE 2007 named late 2009 as the earliest possible date by which Iran could produce enough HEU for a nuclear weapon, it assessed this date to be 'very unlikely', and said that the time frame was more likely to be 2010–2015. It seems that these later dates were posited because of the numerous technical difficulties that Iran encountered before 2008, and the intrinsic flaws in the P-1 centrifuge. Urenco, which developed the machine, never used this first-generation technology for production, and Pakistan abandoned it early on because the machines failed so often. Even if Iran masters the running of P-1-centrifuge cascades in large numbers, the poor quality of the centrifuges may postpone its attainment of the capacity for sustained production of enriched uranium. If Iran were able to produce and operate large numbers of the more efficient second-generation centrifuges that it displayed to the IAEA in January 2008, its ability to produce HEU would be greatly improved and the worst-case time frame might become closer to reality. Iran's progress with advanced

is difficult to predict. The fact that it is continuing to add cascades of exclusively P-1 centrifuges suggests that it is experiencing problems with the new-generation machines. On the other hand, given the improved operational efficiency of the P-1 cascades in 2008, it would not be surprising if the US intelligence community again brought forward its worst-case scenario. Nuclear physicist Richard Garwin stated at the beginning of 2008 that Iran's centrifuges would have to fall far below nominal performance to fail to be able to produce enough HEU for a weapon within a year of the piping at Natanz being reconfigured or 3,000 centrifuges being installed at a hidden location for this purpose.[97] By September, Iran's centrifuges were operating only 15% below the claimed nominal performance.

The timescale for Iranian weapon acquisition is also affected by the weapons designs that could be developed or acquired. Sophisticated weapons with high compression rates can require far smaller amounts of HEU than a standard weapon – as little as 3kg, according to some experts.[98] For a gun-type weapon of the kind that even a small terrorist group could conceivably be capable of building, deliverable in a truck or assembled in a target city, approximately 60kg of HEU would be needed. Notwithstanding the variation in the amount of HEU needed for a weapon, the IAEA's definition of a 'significant quantity' (the amount needed for an implosion device) as 25kg of HEU is still the standard used by most timescale estimates on Iran, although some worst-case analyses posit 15–20kg.

Iran insists that it has no intention to produce HEU, only LEU for reactor fuel. If it did attempt to produce HEU at the safeguarded Natanz facility, IAEA inspectors would know almost immediately. Therefore, if Iran wanted to produce HEU, it would probably do so either in a clandestine facility or by building up a stockpile of LEU, to be further enriched to HEU in a matter of weeks if it chose to withdraw from the NPT. One break-out scenario involves Iran producing a stockpile of LEU under IAEA verification and waiting for one or two years until it has a sufficient quantity before expelling inspectors and enriching the stockpile to weapons grade in five to seven weeks.[99]

The definition of what would make Iran nuclear capable deserves further attention. Having just enough HEU for one implosion device can hardly be said to confer nuclear-weapons status. At a minimum, a state would need two bombs' worth, so that one could be tested. A real deterrent capability would of course require more, in case of device failures and to enable flexibility in war. At its September 2008 rate of production, Iran could produce enough LEU for approximately one weapon a year, once re-enriched to HEU. This timescale could contract if Iran added significantly more centrifuges. On the other hand, Iran might also experience technical problems that would set back production.

Weaponisation

All the timeline estimates assume that if Iran could master the enrichment technology it could also simultaneously learn how to make a weapon out of the HEU thus produced. The timescale for weaponisation is determined by both the type of weapon and the amount of fissile material available. Gun-type weapons are relatively easy to assemble compared with the intricacies of implosion devices but, as noted above, they require much more fissile material, and would be too large for delivery by missile. The timescale also depends on the degree to which there is concern about reliability, predictability and safety. A terrorist group trying to create a crude improvised device might not care about any of these conditions, but the Iranian military presumably would. Among the technical challenges of weaponisation would be the reconfiguring of existing LEU production facilities,[100] or the building of clandestine facilities, the mastery of the HEU production process and the reconversion of HEU to metal, the shaping of the uranium metal into pits, the design of a weapon small enough to fit onto the warhead of a delivery vehicle, the fashioning of the nuclear triggering device and (in the case of implosion devices) of the spherical explosive lenses and reflector, learning how to sustain the nuclear reaction with an additional source of neutrons, and the construction of the device.

All these technical achievements are within Iran's reach. The 2007 NIE judged that 'Iran has the scientific, technical and industrial capacity eventually to produce nuclear weapons if it decides to do so.' Some experts assess that if fissile material were available, even a well-financed sub-national group could construct an implosion weapon in about a year.[101] But several countries that have developed nuclear weapons found that it took longer than they expected. According to the former head of Iraq's nuclear-weapons project, Jafar Dhia Jafar, in 1991, after several years' work on weaponisation, Iraq was still at least three years away from success.[102] A study prepared by the Japanese government in 2006 was reported to have concluded that it would take Japan between three and five years to build a prototype of a miniaturised nuclear warhead, even though Japan already has enrichment and reprocessing plants and an advanced nuclear-science establishment.[103] In both cases, however, it was production of a sufficient quantity of weapons-grade fissile material that was deemed to be the limiting variable.

It is not known how far Iran had progressed in developing nuclear weapons before this work was apparently halted in autumn 2003. Whether the work remains halted is a key intelligence question. CIA Director Michael Hayden said in September 2008 that subsequent intelligence going up to mid 2007 supported the conclusion that Iran had not restarted the weapons programme in that period.[104]

Among other open questions is whether or not Iran received any of the nuclear-weapons-design data that members of the Khan network are known to have stored and copied in electronic form. According to nuclear expert David Albright, computer files that Swiss authorities seized from Swiss nationals Friedrich, Marco and Urs Tinner after the Khan network was rolled up in 2004 contained designs of smaller, more sophisticated nuclear weapons than the Chinese-origin design that the network sold to Libya.[105] Two well-respected reporters have written that Urs Tinner sent computer disks carrying these bomb designs to Khan and his chief lieutenant, B.S.A. Tahir, in early 2004.[106] A senior IAEA official has remarked that other parties are bound also to have received the digitised designs.[107] Western analysts and policymakers must work on the worst-case assumption that Iran was among the recipients of these designs for weapons which, because of their size, would be an ideal fit for *Shahab* missiles.[108]

CHAPTER THREE

Can Iran's Capability Be Kept Non-Weaponised?

Possessing an enrichment capability is not the same as having the Bomb. If enrichment alone conferred weapons status, Japan, Germany, the Netherlands and Brazil would be considered nuclear-weapons capable. All produce enriched uranium for reactor fuel and have the technical capability to convert their industrial-scale facilities to HEU production. With the partial exception of Brazil, however, there is little international concern that any would do so. Their acceptance of IAEA safeguards, history of cooperation with inspections, societal transparency and minimal motivations for proliferating, as well as the economic rationale of their programmes and the absence of any sign of weapons intentions or weapons-related work gives the international community confidence in their non-proliferation bona fides. (Brazil's less-than-perfect record on several of these criteria keeps it on some proliferation watch-lists.)

Iran is viewed differently. On each of the above criteria, Tehran has provided grounds for suspicion, or what ElBaradei has called a 'confidence deficit'.[1] Because its intentions are suspect, its capabilities tend to be judged according to worst-case assumptions. In Iran's case, the line between a nuclear programme for civilian purposes and a military nuclear programme is thin to the point where it is perceived by many to be non-existent. There nevertheless is still a distinction between civilian and military purposes. An oft-cited footnote to the 2007 NIE draws a distinction between Iran's 'declared civil work' on uranium enrichment and 'nuclear weapon design and weaponisation work'.[2] Gareth Evans, president of

Brussels-based conflict-prevention NGO the International Crisis Group, has said that if the world could be confident that the line between civilian and military capability that lies at the heart of the NPT would hold in Iran's case, it would not matter whether the country was capable of producing its own nuclear fuel.[3] The issue is how to build that confidence, and whether it can be built at all while Iran continues enrichment activity.

The problem is that the line is almost invisible. Unless Iran conducts a test, declares itself nuclear-armed or withdraws from the NPT, it will be impossible to judge for certain if and when it has crossed the nuclear threshold. If Iran were to expel inspectors and reconfigure Natanz in an overt break-out, analysts could calculate the number of weeks before a weapon's worth of HEU could be produced using declared facilities. In the more likely case of Iran continuing ostensibly to adhere to the NPT, it would not be possible to know if it were operating clandestine facilities. There are some things that would be clear indicators of a weapons decision, including the discovery of clandestine enrichment, HEU production or weaponisation work, a declaration of weapons status or the unveiling by intelligence of such a status, and testing. However, the common wisdom in the West remains that Iranian possession of nuclear weapons will not be known until after the fact.[4]

Once Iran has the capability, a political decision against weaponisation is the only barrier to it crossing the threshold. The 2007 NIE stated that 'only an Iranian political decision to abandon a nuclear weapons objective would plausibly keep Iran from eventually producing nuclear weapons — and such a decision is inherently reversible'. Iran already has reasons not to cross that line, because of the costs to its security, economy, religious integrity (through what would be a violation of Khamenei's August 2005 fatwa) and regional power. This chapter assesses proposals for making the line between a latent capability and actual weaponisation thicker and more visible.

Fallback proposals

A number of proposals have been made for reducing the risk of Iran crossing the proliferation line. It is widely acknowledged that zero enrichment would be best, but many observers believe that this has become an impossible goal. Since early 2006, Mohamed ElBaradei has argued that the policy focus should be on Iran not enriching on an industrial scale, rather than on the suspension of enrichment activity, on the grounds that the latter goal has been superseded by events and that Iran does not present an imminent threat. Working on the assumption that Iran will never accept zero enrichment and that continuing to demand it is a losing game as the country continues to expand its enrichment capabilities with insufficient safeguards, those who promote fallback proposals favour granting legitimacy to enrichment in Iran in exchange for intrusive inspections.

Most of the fallback proposals would also require limits on the size of Iran's programme, or a delay in it reaching industrial-level size. Their proponents argue that sticking to the current policy of zero enrichment is more likely to produce something close to the worst outcome – an unconstrained, under-safeguarded enrichment capability.[5] Those critical of the current policy also note that time is on Iran's side, as the enrichment programme continues to expand. A senior European official speaking in September 2007 likened sanctions diplomacy to 'a race between how fast they can build centrifuges and we can turn up the pain',[6] to which critics rejoined that 'the centrifuges are winning'.[7] Because capping seems possible but rollback highly improbable, a case can be made for trying to strike a deal before the number of cascades at Natanz grows even larger. An agreement that kept Iran's military nuclear capability latent and lifted the sanctions that impose costs on both sides in the form of lost trade could be characterised as a 'win–win' option.

A 'delayed limited enrichment' plan proposed by the International Crisis Group in February 2006 would have accepted Iranian enrichment in exchange for Tehran suspending the programme for two to three years, then limiting its size to several hundred centrifuges for three to four years while accepting highly intrusive inspections.[8] These limits have been overtaken by the expansion of Iran's programme since they were put forward, but Gareth Evans argues that Iran can still be persuaded to spread its development of industrial-scale enrichment activity over an extended period.[9] In March 2006, Russia reportedly floated a similar proposal whereby, after a period of suspension, Iran would be allowed to undertake 'limited research activities' to supplement a Russian–Iranian joint venture to produce enriched uranium on Russian soil (a venture that Russia first mooted in autumn 2005), while putting off its own industrial-scale enrichment for seven to nine years and granting the IAEA intrusive inspections.[10]

Several proposals by various American and European scholars would offer international support for enrichment in Iran in the form of multinational management and ownership.[11] Since early 2006, MIT physicist Geoffrey Forden and former UK Ambassador to the UN John Thomson have advocated that an international consortium be established in partnership with Iran to lease all Iranian facilities connected with enrichment and to lease advanced Urenco centrifuges for production of fuel in Iran for export to the surrounding region.[12] The concept of multinational owner-ship picked up momentum in 2008 when it was promoted by former US Ambassadors William Luers and Thomas Pickering and MIT scholar Jim Walsh.[13] Matthew Bunn of Harvard combines two approaches in arguing that a limited number of centrifuge cascades operated by international staff is the option with the most tolerable risk.[14] Among other conditions, the proposals outlined above would variously require that Iran not conduct any work on nuclear fuel outside the multilateral arrangement, that production of HEU (or LEU above 5%) and plutonium reprocessing not be undertaken, that Iran use only light-water reactors and that the treaty establishing the consortium not have a withdrawal clause.

A number of the proposals that have come out of America and Europe include ingenious technical methods for blocking proliferation pathways. Suggestions include requiring that enriched uranium either be stored outside Iran or immediately converted into fuel rods so that it cannot easily be re-enriched to HEU (the latter being a measure that Iran itself suggested); that the enrichment technology leased by any international consortium be 'black-boxed', that is, encased in a way that would keep the technology unavailable to Iranian nationals; that the ball-bearing mecha-nisms of the centrifuges be equipped with a self-destructive device that is automatically triggered in the event of unauthorised use; and that all facili-ties be required to be above ground and not in hardened shelters, so that they may be easily destroyed by air strikes in response to Iranian seizure of the facility in a break-out scenario.

Iran has repeatedly voiced its support for an international consortium – and even proposed a version of the idea itself – on condition that the enrichment takes place on Iranian soil. In a September 2005 speech to the United Nations, Ahmadinejad said that Iran was 'prepared to engage in serious partnership with private and public sectors of other countries in the implementation of a uranium enrichment program in Iran'.[15] In July 2007 talks with Javier Solana, Ali Larijani made the case for an international nuclear consortium, which he claimed Solana initially welcomed but later rejected.[16] In February 2008, Ahmadinejad said that Iran's proposal was 'no longer on the table. But if others formulated it again, we would study it – under one condition: that the Iranian people's right to enrich uranium be preserved.'[17] In May 2008, Iran formally tabled with UN Secretary-General Ban Ki-moon a negotiation proposal calling for the establishment of 'enrichment and nuclear fuel production consortiums in different parts of the world – including in Iran'.[18]

Would Iran accept conditions that prevented break-out?

Technical solutions will not solve the problem, however, unless Iran makes a strategic decision not to seek a nuclear-weapons capability. In purely technical terms, it is possible to devise satisfactory ways of strengthening the line separating a non-weaponised capability from weapons manufacture. Although the line cannot be made impermeable and some of the ideas that have been put forward suffer from excessive optimism, the main problem is not technical feasibility. If Iran's centrifuge programme truly could be limited to 3,000–4,000 P-1 centrifuges that did not work well and tended to break down, ElBaradei would be correct that it would not present an imminent proliferation threat. The threat would be further diminished if the operation of the cascades was also limited in terms of the UF_6 feed rate and hours of operation, keeping the centrifuges from enriching continuously. It would be naïve, however, to assume that Iran would stop there, and not work secretly on the more advanced centrifuges and gradually push beyond any limits imposed.

Lack of confidence in Iran's intentions is the central problem. As discussed in Chapter 1, there are compelling reasons to believe that the principal purpose of Iran's enrichment programme is to create a nuclear-weapons capability. If this is the case, then no technical solution will work, because Iran will not accept any condition that would prevent it from attaining this objective.[19] Iran may well accept the general notion of an international consortium. But in the event that such a plan were formally proposed and negotiations held over its details, it seems clear that Iran would not accept the kinds of limits on the programme and Security Council enforcement powers that the major powers would require to guard against the possibility of NPT break-out. Iran will not accept the kind of intrusive inspections that were forced on Iraq in 1991. Blanket restrictions on Iranian access to technology, such as the black-boxing condition mentioned above, would be rejected as violating inalienable rights and Iran's core goal of achieving and demonstrating technical proficiency. The low probability of Iran ceding control of its nuclear programme to the international community is even lower now that the country has demonstrated an enrichment capability. In its official statements about accepting multilateral facilities, Iran has not said that it would put its own facilities under multinational control.[20] It can be expected that other proposed restrictions would be neither accepted nor rejected, but would effectively be shunted aside through non-responsive counter-proposals and endless negotiation and filibuster, which was how Iran dealt with both Russia's 2005 proposal for a joint uranium-enrichment venture on Russian soil and the E3+3 proposal of June 2008.

Meanwhile, taking a fallback position that accepted enrichment in Iran would incur the immediate cost of establishing a new negotiation benchmark. By proposing a fallback option, the E3+3 would be conceding its goal of no enrichment and offering legitimacy to an activity that it had hitherto judged to be unacceptable and that the UN Security Council had mandated be suspended. Securing international recognition of a right to enrichment has been a major goal for Iran. Before granting this concession, it would be appropriate to receive a concession of equivalent value in return, ideally one that is equally irreversible. Once Iran's enrichment programme was accepted as legitimate, the concession could not be retrieved in the event that negotiations broke down. Iran's claim to a right to enrichment could no longer be legitimately questioned unless the country committed new safeguards violations.

Furthermore, Iran does not claim this right for some philosophical purpose, but rather to use it. Legitimising the programme would also have the effect of legitimising Iran's course of action to date. These and other costs of fallback options are outlined in more detail below.

'Testing Iran's intentions'

It is sometimes argued that offering a fallback position would at least test Iran's intentions, and that, in the event that Iran rejected technical solutions, the US would be better placed to garner international support for coercive action.[21] Such arguments for why the US should be willing to offer concessions have been made at each stage of the European-led engagement strategy. It is true that US concessions in the direction of greater engagement with Iran brought Europeans, and to a lesser extent Russia and China, into closer conformity with US policy on sanctions. Such concessions have not had any impact on Iran's basic stance, however. Since 2005, Tehran's intentions have repeatedly been tested by a number of US compromises, listed opposite. In the words of Middle East analyst Ray Takeyh – an advocate of détente with Iran – 'it's been slow-motion capitulation since 2005'.[22] During the same period, Iran, which had previously made several compromises of its own, has become increasingly unbending.

If the US and its allies make the further concession of legitimising Iran's enrichment programme and Iran then crosses the line anyway, the ability of Western capitals to influence the international community will have suffered for their having shown misplaced confidence in Iran's intentions.[23] Given Iran's long history of safeguards violations and unsatisfactory cooperation with the IAEA, there is ample reason to be sceptical about those intentions.

US compromises and policy changes 2005–08

- **March 2005:** President Bush announces his support for European negotiations with Iran.

- **March 2005:** US offers to remove veto on Iran joining WTO and allow sale of parts for commercial aircraft. (The WTO veto is removed in May. An expedited sale of engine spare parts for Airbus jetliners operated by Iran Air is approved in September 2006.)

- **June 2005:** Secretary of State Rice acknowledges Iran's right to civil nuclear energy.

- **November 2005:** US accept UF_6 conversion in Iran, in connection with Russian proposal for joint venture to enrich uranium in Russia.

- **May 2006:** US agrees to join talks with Iran and take part in the E3+3 offer of incentives, which include sale of nuclear technology.

- **June 2006:** In E3+3 offer, US agrees that enrichment moratorium could be reviewed once IAEA has confirmed that all outstanding issues and concerns are resolved and international confidence in the exclusively peaceful nature of Iran's civil nuclear programme has been restored.

- **January 2007:** Rice expresses willingness to meet Iranian leadership 'anytime, anywhere' to discuss any subject, as long as Iran suspends enrichment.

- **May 2007:** US agrees to E3+3 offer to accept cap on the number of centrifuges (the 'double freeze') in place of a full suspension, as condition for initiating 'pre-negotiations'.

- **June 2008:** In repackaged E3+3 proposal, US agrees that Iranian nuclear R&D could continue 'as confidence was gradually restored', and nods in the direction of security assurances with an expression of its willingness to 'reaffirm [its] obligations' under the UN Charter to refrain from threat or use of force.

- **July 2008:** US floats prospect of posting diplomats to US interests section in Tehran.

- **July 2008:** US sends State Department Under Secretary William Burns to join E3+3 'pre-negotiations' with Iran in Geneva, despite no suspension or capping.

Iran's negotiating 'flexibility'

It is sometimes argued that if the West had been willing at an earlier date to compromise on the central issue and accept the principle of enrichment on Iranian soil, the programme could have been kept at a far lower level than is possible today. In November 2004, for example, when Iran was negotiating the Paris Agreement on suspension, it sought an allowance to continue R&D with only 20 centrifuges. In spring 2005, Iran indicated that if a 64-centrifuge pilot cascade were accepted, industrial-scale enrichment could be put off for ten years.[24] As Iran's capabilities improve, the ante for any potential deal on limits will keep on increasing. The proposition that a deal should have been struck while the iron was hot cannot be proven, however, because there is no way of knowing if Iran would have agreed to any deal that set long-term limits. Had such a deal been reached, it is another question as to whether Iran would have agreed on a shared interpretation and not sought to adjust the limits. Judging by Iran's negotiating style and historical record, it appears more likely that as Iran perfected the operation of smaller cascades, it would have increased centrifuge numbers and sought to renegotiate based on the new facts on the ground. Iran has never offered to limit its enrichment programme to a size smaller than its size at the time of negotiation, and second-hand suggestions for limits on the programme made by unofficial interlocutors have always been pitched somewhere above the level already attained.

As argued above, so long as Iran's intention is to acquire a weapons break-out capability, it will not accept terms that prevent it from achieving this goal. The history of the October 2003 Tehran Agreement on suspension, the terms of which Iran repeatedly redefined and renegotiated, is instructive in this regard. It is also instructive to recall the justification of the agreement that was offered to a domestic audience by former chief negotiator Hassan Rowhani – that Iran had agreed to suspend activities only in areas in which it did not have technical problems, and that in the calm diplomatic environment of the suspension, Iran would be able to complete work on the uranium-conversion process.[25]

Evidence of some debate within Iran notwithstanding, the country's willingness to compromise, or even negotiate, has decreased even as external pressure on it to do so has increased. The enrichment programme has become ingrained in Iranian national consciousness as a 'right' that cannot be circumscribed. Given the extraordinarily high level of popular support that the programme commands (81% of those polled in a February–March 2008 survey considered it 'very important' for Iran to have a full nuclear fuel cycle[26]), it is difficult to envisage Iran accepting any solution that does not involve enrichment continuing in some form on Iranian soil. The country's negotiating flexibility is also constrained by Ayatollah Khamenei's entrenched view that any compromise with the US will only be met with demands for additional compromises.[27]

Intrusive inspections and CTBT ratification

In May 2008, President Ahmadinejad claimed that Iran would not accept even the Additional Protocol as long as Israel remained outside the NPT.[28] This was a harder line on inspections than Iran had taken hitherto. Whether it was adopted only for propaganda purposes is unclear. Iran had in the recent past emphasised that if its enrichment activities were accepted, it would accept more intrusive inspections, including implementation of the Additional Protocol and a continuous on-site presence of IAEA inspectors at Natanz and Esfahan.[29] Such measures could have some merit, but would not be sufficient to detect undeclared nuclear activities elsewhere. For this purpose, much more intrusive IAEA monitoring is needed. The agency's knowledge of Iran's enrichment programme has steadily declined since

Iran closed off inspection of centrifuge-manufacturing sites in February 2006 and subsequently rescinded a provision of its safeguards agreement which required it to provide design information to the IAEA before constructing any new nuclear facilities.[30] Improved IAEA monitoring would give greater notice of weapons-related work, help to deter Iranian cheating and reduce the danger of over-reaction by the US and Israel on the basis of worst-case assumptions. Many observers therefore argue for accepting an 'enrichment for transparency' trade.[31]

The concept of an intrusive inspection regime is often referred to in shorthand as 'Additional Protocol Plus' as, for example, in the recommendations of a high-level IAEA commission published in May 2008.[32] The term is open to interpretation – and misinterpretation – because there is no established standard for what the 'plus' should be. In the case of Iran it should include, at a minimum, the transparency measures that were called for by ElBaradei in a September 2005 report subsequently endorsed by the IAEA Board of Governors: 'access to individuals, documentation related to procurement, dual use equipment, certain military owned workshops and research and development locations'.[33]

For any state found to be non-compliant with its safeguards agreement as Iran has been, former head of the IAEA's Safeguards Department Pierre Goldschmidt suggests a more comprehensive set of additional IAEA inspection rights. These include prompt access to persons involved in the programme, broader and prompter access to locations where nuclear-related activity may be taking place, in-situ access to original data and documents and copies thereof, broader and faster access to information (including answers to questions and challenges about inconsistencies), the entitlement to wide-area environmental sampling and use of any recording or measurement devices deemed appropriate by the agency, and no arbitrary restrictions on the selection of agency inspectors. To provide these inspection rights, he recommends that the Security Council adopt a generic resolution to automatically apply a 'Temporary Complementary Protocol' to each state in non-compliance until the IAEA is able to conclude that there is no undeclared nuclear material or activities in the state and that its declarations to the agency are correct and complete.[34]

Beyond intrusive inspections, it would be useful to persuade Iran to ratify the Comprehensive Nuclear Test Ban Treaty (CTBT), which it signed in 1996. Although Iran's history of safeguards violations gives no reassurance that it would not violate or withdraw from a CTBT, ratification by Iran (one of the eight remaining states whose ratification is required for entry into force of the treaty) would create an additional legal and symbolic barrier to overt weapons status. It would also be a practical barrier, to the extent that even if Iran obtained a proven test design from the Khan network, it could not be sure that an implosion bomb would work without a test. Iran voices no unalterable objections to CTBT ratification, but takes cover behind the refusal of Egypt, Israel, China and the US to ratify. US ratification would remove an excuse for continuing to hold out.

Might non-weaponised deterrence be enough for Iran?

It is possible that Iran does not need to actually assemble or test nuclear weapons in order to achieve the strategic, political and psychological benefits of being seen to have a nuclear-weapons capability. Deterrence has much to do with perception. Mastery of the technology should satisfy the national-prestige imperative and be sufficient for most of Iran's deterrence needs, without the security costs, economic sanctions and political ostracism that would be forthcoming if Iran visibly crossed the line. Iranians of all political stripes have made this case,[35] although the argument is not very reassuring to outsiders, given the weapons-development work that Iran kept up from the late 1980s to 2003. The unsavoury prospect of Iran using a nuclear-capable status for regional hegemony and blackmail is one reason the West hopes to deny Iran full mastery of enrichment technology. In terms of the danger of break-out, it matters a great deal whether the 'programme-in-being' is akin more to that of Japan or Israel, the two extremes along the scale from complete transparency to complete opacity. Despite its break-out capability, Japan enjoys widespread international confidence in its non-proliferation bona fides, whereas Israel is assumed to possess 100–200 weapons with sophisticated designs. Iran's transparency is somewhere in the middle, while its intentions appear to be closer to the Israeli model.

Assessing the risks

Fallback options should be assessed in terms of their feasibility and their likely impact on various proliferation risks. These are: 1) the risk of diversion of nuclear material and knowledge; 2) the risk of clandestine development; 3) the risk of NPT break-out; and 4) the risk of proliferation elsewhere in the region and beyond.

Risk of diversion

Diversion of nuclear material (that is, LEU, plus unenriched UF_6 feedstock and some earlier conversion products) is the least worrying of the risks. Standard IAEA safeguards are designed to detect and thereby deter the diversion of material from declared facilities. As long as Iran adheres to its Comprehensive Safeguards Agreement, the IAEA's material accounting techniques can adequately protect against diversion from small to medium-sized facilities such as Natanz. Whether such safeguards can prevent diversion from very large enrichment facilities is debatable, given the amount of material that would be unaccounted for due to uncertainties inherent in measurement systems and the accumulation of material in piping. This would be of particular concern for fallback schemes such as the Forden–Thomson plan for large-scale enrichment in Iran for export purposes. Advocates of such plans argue that Iran would need to be willing to run a very large risk of detection to try to divert material from safeguarded facilities, and that the stronger the verification effort, the less likely the possibility of diversion.[36]

Risk of clandestine development
A far greater risk than diversion of material from safeguarded facilities is that Iran might produce HEU secretly using feed material produced clandestinely. There is concern that, after mastering the technology of running an enrichment cascade, Iran could replicate this capability at facilities unreported to the IAEA. Such facilities would require both physical resources (enrichment-related equipment and uranium) and technical knowledge. The 2007 NIE judged that Iran would probably use covert facilities rather than declared sites for any HEU production, and noted growing indications that Iran had been engaged in covert uranium-conversion and enrichment activity. It also judged, however, that these efforts were probably halted in 2003, along with weaponisation efforts. It would be logical for Iran to have prepared alternative enrichment facilities for use in the event that Natanz is bombed, or at least to have plans for such facilities. If such a clandestine facility did exist, it would also be logical to install some centrifuges in it, or else to keep a quantity of machines hidden for post-bombing reconstitution of an enrichment programme. However, Iran appears to be following the alternative approach of constructing and installing as many centrifuges as it can in the declared facility at Natanz.[37] Under the intrusive inspection regime that would have to accompany any fallback option, all centrifuges and their components would need to be safeguarded. In addition to UF_6 feed material, all intermediary conversion products, as well as uranium mines and, ideally, yellowcake, would also be safeguarded. This would make the diversion of physical resources to a clandestine plant more difficult.

Diversion of knowledge is harder to prevent. Centrifuge designs and documents concerning centrifuge-cascade operation can be kept under lock and key, but not so the technical knowledge residing in the heads of trained personnel. Although it is true that many of the measures proposed by consortium advocates could do a better job of protecting against technology diversion than the safeguards that are presently applied in Iran, multinational consortium schemes that involved the transfer of knowledge to Iran would increase the risk of know-how later being diverted to unsafeguarded facilities. If a multilateral facility operated centrifuges that were already in Iran's inventory, the tacit knowledge gained on the shop floor of the facility would be directly applicable to indigenous efforts. If the multilateral facility operated more advanced centrifuges, the tacit knowledge would probably be less applicable to any clandestine machinery, but the risk of boosting Iran's HEU-production capability would be greater in the event of the facilities being expropriated.

Clandestine development is more difficult to detect if Iran is able to operate legitimate enrichment facilities than if any such activity is a violation of Security Council resolutions. From a technical standpoint, an authorised operation may mask signals from a clandestine programme.[38] From a legal perspective, legitimising even a low level of enrichment would make it impossible for inspectors to prove that any evidence they found of centrifuge-component production was for clandestine purposes and not part of the replacement cycle for the acknowledged programme. Legitimising the programme would also undermine the ability of Western allies to block Iran's foreign-procurement effort. A tight international export-control system is the best means of impeding Iran's ability to produce fissile material. If enrichment activity were legitimised, these controls would inevitably weaken and Iran would be able to hide all purchases behind the mask of the authorised programme.[39]

Proponents of plans for multinational enrichment facilities counter that the technical know-how that Iran would gain would be more than offset by the enhanced inspection procedures that would be applied and the additional value of what Forden and Thomson call 'social monitoring mechanisms' – having international personnel on site with 'eyes on the ground'.[40] International personnel working at the facilities – at every stage of the enrichment process, in the most robust proposals – would get to know all the significant Iranian technicians and engineers and thus be aware of any unexplained absences that might indicate diversion of knowledge to a clandestine programme. International personnel could also supplement formal inspections by investigating any suspicious activity. Combined with the Additional Protocol and other intrusive measures, as well as conditions that prohibited any sensitive fuel-cycle activity outside the confines of the multinational programme and that black-boxed the leased foreign technology, this additional layer of 'societal' safeguards would in theory increase the level of confidence in the absence of unde-clared nuclear facilities or activities. By being on the ground constantly and having more direct material-accountancy information, the multilateral plant operators would be able to offer more timely detection of diversion than could be provided by periodic IAEA audits.

Societal controls have their limits, however. Iran could to a large extent evade such controls by giving cascade-operation training to newly-minted nuclear physics graduates unknown to the international managers. Opportunities for technical diversion could grow as Iranian staff developed greater technical proficiency.[41] Proponents of multilateral consortia reply that Iran may learn more advanced enrichment tech-niques anyway, and that enrichment technologies alone are not sufficient to manufacture a nuclear weapon. These counter-arguments have techni-cal merit, but they are not persuasive. Even if intrusive inspections and societal monitoring minimised the risk of parallel clandestine operations to which technical know-how could be diverted, no inspection regime can protect against the risk of personnel being re-employed in an NPT break-out scenario.

Risk of NPT break-out

Any option that involves Iran operating enrichment facilities carries the risk that these could be used to contribute to HEU production in the event of withdrawal from the NPT. The risk increases if Iran is able to build up a stockpile of LEU. By starting with LEU rather than natural uranium, Iran could reduce by a factor of four the time needed to produce HEU of weapons grade. Under the status quo, the risk of break-out increases with each day that Iran installs new centrifuges, improves cascade opera-tion and stockpiles LEU. Fallback options for limiting such expansion may deserve consideration, although it remains doubtful that limits would be effective. Options that would provide Iran with additional technology that could be seized in a break-out scenario would exacerbate the danger. In a country that has expropriated foreign assets in the past and that still holds to revolutionary ideals, the possibility of seizure of multilateral enrich-ment equipment cannot be discounted.

Proponents of fallback options have suggested various conditions that would in principle reduce the risk of break-out, including the requirement that all LEU produced be stored outside the country. Arrangements for a multilateral enrichment facility could be structured to build political and commercial protection against break-out. Foreign customers of the facility would bring pressure to bear on Iran not to do anything that would jeopardise their fuel supply, and there would be no withdrawal clause in the contract. Unilateral abrogation of the agreement and nationalisation of the facilities – in effect, the expropriation of others' property – would signal an end to peaceful intentions and thereby trigger severe consequences, including military action.[42]

This last argument, however, appears to place undue trust in an international system that did not prove able to take effective action to stop North Korea's nuclear-weapons programme after it expelled inspectors and abrogated the Agreed Framework in 2003. Faith in swift and severe international responses in the event of Iranian treaty violations should also be shaken by the international community's delayed and ineffectual response to the IAEA's 2003 uncovering of systematic safeguards violations in Iran, whereby it took two and a half years to bring the case to the Security Council and almost another year to adopt the first sanctions. In a break-out scenario, Iran could produce enough HEU for a weapon in a matter of a few months, if not weeks. Given the apparent military purpose of Iran's enrichment programme, the country's leadership is unlikely to accept conditions on any fallback option that would preclude the achievement of this capability. And given Iran's record on hostage-taking,[43] there is also the risk that, in a break-out, Iran might hold Western technicians hostage in the facilities to try to deter air strikes.

The hope behind the multilateral enrichment facility idea is that it might stimulate a reframing of the incentives that drive the nuclear programme. The appeal of ongoing access to Western technology could conceivably give the Atomic Energy Organisation of Iran an incentive to argue internally against clandestine development and break-out options.[44] It has also been suggested that an offer of international support for a peaceful nuclear programme and the lifting of sanctions could give reformists or pragmatic conservatives in Iran a persuasive new narrative with which to counter the nuclear nationalism that has been central to Ahmadinejad's appeal.[45] Such arguments rest, however, on the doubtful assumption that Ahmadinejad's opponents do not themselves support the goal of a weapons capability or could be induced to argue against it in internal discussions. It was, after all, Hashemi Rafsanjani, Ahmadinejad's opponent in the 2005 presidential race, who in 2001 spoke of winning a nuclear exchange with Israel.[46] And it was under the reformist Khatami administration that the enrichment programme accelerated. Accepting an enrichment programme in Iran would give Ahmadinejad a propaganda victory by allowing him to claim the vindication of his hardline posture. Rather than encouraging moderation, it could encourage further defiance.

Feasibility questions

More foreign personnel on the ground would certainly be an improvement on the minimal IAEA monitoring that Iran allows today. It is not realistic, however, to assume that Iran would agree to tight constraints on its enrichment activity, unless the country's leadership had made a strategic policy decision not to seek a latent weapons capability. Although the leadership expresses interest in multinational-consortium ideas, it shows little willingness to give up management and control of its national programme. In the event that Iran did agree to international control of a facility or to limits on the extent of the enrichment programme, Western leaders could have no confidence that the deal would be honoured in practice without 'salami-slicing' gradual encroachments on agreed limits. Iran's past form, notably its behaviour in the aftermath of the October 2003 suspension agreement, gives cause for concern that once its technicians were able to surmount the technical problems associated with a legitimised small-scale programme, Iran would break any such deal, first with small infractions and by exploiting loopholes, and eventually by moving on to larger-scale production.

Other feasibility issues arise with regard to the specifics of various anti-proliferation precautions. While the black-boxing of enrichment technology may be sufficient to protect commercial secrets when the partners in question are France or the US, for example, it is more difficult to protect secrets in a hostile environment where it is national policy to acquire weapons-useful technology. Furthermore, the social bonds that would naturally develop between foreign experts and local staff at a multilateral facility could well lead to a leaking of technology secrets. Relying on self-destructive devices to render centrifuges inoperative in the event of unauthorised use assumes that Iran would not be able to engineer countermeasures. Such optimism may be misplaced. There is also the question of whether self-destruct techniques would even be applicable in practice, given the danger that could be posed to plant personnel.

Risk of stimulating a proliferation cascade

How the Iranian nuclear problem evolves will inevitably have repercussions elsewhere. Tehran's programme has already created the potential for a nuclear-proliferation cascade in the surrounding region. Several of the 13 countries in the greater Middle East that between February 2006 and January 2007 announced an intention to explore nuclear energy were spurred, at least in part, by a political or security imperative to keep pace with Iran.[47] If Iran's enrichment efforts succeed, and a once-unacceptable situation is accepted, others could be emboldened to go the same route, or at least to start by establishing nuclear-power programmes and keeping open the option of pursuing sensitive technologies. Acknowledging an Iranian right to enrichment as part of a strategy to limit Iranian proliferation thus could have the perverse effect of encouraging proliferation elsewhere. Legitimisation of the Iranian programme could increase the security motivations of Iran's neighbours for seeking such a programme themselves, and give them reason to believe that the US, even if it initially opposed the expansion of sensitive fuel-cycle technology, would eventually accept their nuclear plans as well, even if, as in Iran's case, there was no economic rationale for them.

Other than Iran and Israel, no country in the greater Middle East region is known today to seek sensitive fuel-cycle capabilities, and at least three (Bahrain, Saudi Arabia and the UAE) have explicitly said that they would not seek indigenous enrichment or reprocessing facilities. Elsewhere in the region, however, intentions are less clear. Egypt, which has explored nuclear weapons in the past, insists that it will not rule out sensitive technologies nor accept further non-proliferation controls as long as Israel remains outside the NPT. Algeria, which reportedly possesses a dormant reprocessing plant, appears to have the same attitude. Until September 2007, Syria was building a plutonium-production reactor for highly suspect purposes. Turkey has denied press reports that it seeks enrichment, but has both the technological capability and the political motivation to keep parity with Iran. These latter four countries are all potential candidates for joining a proliferation cascade, as is Saudi Arabia, although it would be more likely to pursue a nuclear deterrent by purchasing weapons than through indigenous development.[48]

As long as Iran remains under increasing pressure to stop its sensitive nuclear activities and is penalised for failing to do so, its neighbours have a disincentive against seeking enrichment or reprocessing capabilities of their own. Any fallback option that legitimised Iran's enrichment efforts would diminish that disincentive. By contrast, strategies that strengthened the barriers to military nuclear capabilities would relax proliferation pressures in the region by reducing the uncertainty about covert facilities and break-out capabilities.

In addition to its implications for the Middle East, the outcome of the Iran nuclear crisis will have an important impact on the global non-proliferation regime. Faith in the non-proliferation regime will be under-mined if the international community is unable to dissuade or prevent Iran from developing nuclear-weapons capabilities. Proponents of a multilateral-enrichment solution to the Iranian nuclear problem argue that a multilateral arrangement in Iran could help the regime by provid-ing a model for dealing with the more general global problem of how to stop the spread of indigenous enrichment and reprocessing programmes.[49] International control of enrichment and reprocessing facilities is precisely the solution to this broader problem that ElBaradei and others have advo-cated. Winning the right to enrichment and international support for a national nuclear programme after successfully defying the demands of the Security Council and the IAEA Board, however, is hardly a model one would wish to see emulated. A better precedent is set by creating norms against the expansion of sensitive fuel-cycle technology that is unneces-sary and uneconomical.

Further disadvantages of fallback options
Fallback options would confer legitimacy on an enrichment programme that the Security Council had, after great effort, officially delegitimised, unanimously and with successive reinforcement in the form of four Chapter VII resolutions. Once conferred, this legitimacy would not be reversible, and even to make the offer would be to acknowledge the right to enrichment. Under a fallback deal, Security Council sanctions would fall away and international enterprises would resume business with Iran. The reimposition of financial pressure if Iran reneged on an agreement would be neither certain nor quick.[50] The undermining of the logic and authority of the five Security Council resolutions to date that mandated full suspen-sion is not an insignificant price to pay for an uncertain bet on a fallback scenario. Pierre Goldschmidt notes that without the Security Council requirement for full suspension under Chapter VII, it would not be illegal for Iran to produce weapons-grade HEU, even if there were no apparent civilian use for it. In the event of a fallback scenario, the Council would thus need at a minimum to specify the limits of the allowable enrichment capacity and the corresponding activity, but agreeing on such limits would be a time-consuming task.[51]

Working out the complex legal, financial and technical issues involved in setting up a new multinational enrichment arrangement in Iran would also present huge challenges.[52] Not least of these is the practical problem of persuading foreign companies to enter into a venture with such obvious economic, security and political risks. In an industry in which personnel resources are already stretched to meet the growing demands of a nuclear-energy renaissance, it would not be easy to find experienced engineers prepared to work in an environment in which they would be expected to perform intelligence duties and work under the multiple personal security risks of self-destructive centrifuges, air strikes and hostage-taking. The market solution of providing sufficient remuneration to attract qualified personnel raises the additional question of who would cover the costs of what is likely to be an uneconomical venture. No Western company has any interest in the idea. Finally, there is the question of the political viability of engaging in such cooperation with a state that supplies explosives to militants to kill US and British forces in Iraq and has reportedly aided the Taliban to this purpose in Afghanistan, not to mention its support for violence against Israel and denial of that country's right to exist. The nuclear threat is the most important issue regarding Iran, but it cannot be viewed in isolation.

CONCLUSION

Claims that the West's current policy is highly likely to lead to an unconstrained Iranian enrichment programme are unduly pessimistic. Notwithstanding the progress that Iran has made to date, concerned countries can still restrict Iran's fissile-material-production capability through export controls, sanctions and other means. Only a limited number of high-tech firms manufacture the parts and materials that Iran cannot produce by itself, and Iranian access to these foreign goods is being tightly controlled. Although Iran has in the past acquired enough materials for perhaps up to 10,000 P-1 centrifuges,[1] it cannot be assumed that expansion is unlimited or that Iran is self-sufficient in all areas of centrifuge-enrichment technology. Export controls and sanctions are unlikely to prevent Iran from acquiring a nuclear-weapons capability, but they can limit and delay the programme. The intelligence challenge for the West is to find and exploit the areas in which Iran's programme remains vulnerable.

One vulnerability is Iran's inability so far to produce and operate significant numbers of advanced-generation centrifuges. If Iran had sufficient parts for its advanced-generation machines, it would not continue to install additional cascades of the crash-prone, inefficient P-1 model (unless it has been installing the advanced machines in a clandestine facility). It is important to restrict the programme before Iran is able to make a breakthrough to using an advanced-generation model in large numbers. The need to restrict Iran's freedom to perfect advanced models is another reason to be wary of granting legitimacy to the enrichment programme.

It is also why any agreement on suspension should include suspension of centrifuge research and development work.

The intelligence assessment that Iran made a choice in 2003 to suspend enrichment activity and work on weaponisation gives reason to believe that the suspension called for in the Security Council resolutions may still be possible, despite Iran's rejection of this demand to date. Knowing why Iran decided to stop the weaponisation programme in 2003 would help the West to devise strategies for keeping the country's weapons capabilities latent. The constellation of factors that prevailed in 2003 was unique in terms of both the various forms of pressure brought to bear on Iran and the presence of a government willing to give priority to trade and economics. Since that time, national pride has underpinned Iran's insistence that it can never suspend its progress again. But the possibility cannot be ruled out that a different set of leaders in Tehran might take a position that better serves the country's economic interests.

For now, the best strategy is to maintain the binary choice put to Iran since 2005: international integration, with foreign cooperation on state-of-the-art nuclear-power projects and guaranteed supply of sensitive fuel-cycle services; or political and economic isolation as the price of persisting with indigenous enrichment and plutonium production. The alternative pathway open to Iran is illuminated by the various French and American nuclear-cooperation agreements with Arab countries that accept fuel-cycle services from abroad. It seems probable that, at least in the near term, Iran will stick with the go-it-alone path. Predictions further out are less clear. If the factional power balance in Tehran shifts toward pragmatists willing to negotiate, the balance for the E3+3 between the pros and cons of seeking a compromise could shift. In the meantime, the current supply-side strategy, with some tactical adjustments – including direct US engagement with Iran – is the 'least bad' way of minimising the proliferation risk. Maintaining Security Council sanctions, financial pressure, strict national export controls and international vigilance presents the best hope of keeping Iran's fissile-material-production capability limited in scale and effectiveness. As advocated below, strengthening the pressure that states can bring to bear outside the Security Council creates leverage for the E3+3 in future negotiations, when compromise can be approached from a position of strength. The combination of pressures also serves as a disincentive to other states to follow Iran's path.

For the time being, it is not necessary to strengthen the positive side of the binary choice. The inducements offered to Iran are already substantial and clear. Debates over how to further increase incentives add to the carpet-dealer dynamic that gives Iran reason to wait to see how the Western offer will improve. Non-proliferation analyst George Perkovich makes an intriguing suggestion that the E3+3 should give Iran one last chance to negotiate and if the answer is again negative then they should withdraw the proffered incentives on the grounds that Iran has already achieved the capability that the original inducements were intended to forestall.[2]

Future negotiations

If future Iranian leaders show a willingness to negotiate, the incentives package can be retabled. The US has many potential incentive cards to play in future negotiations, including allowing direct flight connections between the US and Tehran, the release of impounded Iranian funds (amounting to around $10bn) and the lifting of sanctions imposed since 1979. Alone, however, tangible incentives such as these do not appear to affect the motivations behind Iran's enrichment programme. If Iran is ever to be persuaded to forgo sensitive fuel-cycle technologies, some substitute will be needed for the prestige and security benefits that Iranian leaders believe they derive from the enrichment programme.

Iran's negotiating partners should base their position on what they want and let Iran do its own negotiating. Further incentives need not be offered up front. As a matter of analysis, however, the negotiators should try to anticipate the other side's requirements. In the collective judgement of participants in a Brookings Institution working group in spring 2008, for Iran, these include: an end to international isolation and sanctions; acknowledgment of Iran's sovereignty and regional role; a security guarantee from the US; and an end to US-funded democracy-promotion efforts.[3] Engaging with Iran need not equate with recognising the Islamic Republic, which could be a card to play in exchange for specific Iranian actions once negotiations commence. The US has been willing to put such cards in play in dealing with the other major proliferation problem case, engaging bilaterally with North Korea on an unofficial basis and in the format of multilateral talks formally respecting the sovereignty of the Democratic People's Republic of Korea, affirming no intention to attack or invade the country, and committing to moving forward to full diplomatic relations.

Security guarantees

Security guarantees are often assumed to be a necessary part of any solution,[4] and in private, Iranians frequently speak of a need for tangible assurances against US-led 'regime change'. Publicly, however, Iran's current leaders claim not to seek any such guarantees. For example, in a July 2007 interview with a German magazine, Ali Larijani repeated the standard Iranian position that 'We do not need any security guarantees on the part of the USA.'[5] An editorialist for the hardline *Keyhan* newspaper recently wrote that:

> Iran does not have 'security expectations' and therefore Iran is not prepared to abandon its programme in return for any such security assurances ... On the contrary, Iran primarily believes that there is no such thing as American 'security reassurances' which can be trusted; secondly, Iran does not require security reassurances from America.[6]

Several scholars argue that, on this point, Iran means what it says. Ray Takeyh contends that 'the guardians of the theocratic regime do not fear the United States; they do not relate to the international community from a position of strategic vulnerability. Tehran now seeks not assurances against US military strikes but an acknowledgment of its status and influence.'[7] Other knowledgeable observers, such as Columbia University's Gary Sick, reply that Iran naturally will not ask for security guarantees, because to do so would be a sign of weakness.[8]

While Ahmadinejad's administration may not seek security guarantees, the negotiating team under his predecessor made clear their security concerns. In January 2005, an eight-page Iranian proposal to the E3 began with a statement of the principles of 'respect for each other's sovereign equality' and 'rejection of any threat or use of force against each other's national sovereignty, territorial integrity or political independence' and the inviolability of their respective international borders. In July 2004 meetings with E3 representatives in Paris, Iran requested that the addressing of its 'security concerns' be among the conditions for agreeing to consider a temporary suspension of its fuel-cycle programme.[9] In May 2003, in an unanswered proposal for comprehensive negotiations sent to Washington through Swiss Ambassador to Tehran Tim Guldimann, Iran listed six requests, the first of which was for a 'halt [to] US hostile behaviour and rectifications [sic] of status of Iran in the US'. In parenthesis, this was explained as 'interference in internal or external relations, "axis of evil", terrorism list'. Among the five other points was a request for 'recognition of Iran's legitimate security interests in the region'.[10]

For there to be a satisfactory solution to the nuclear crisis, Iran's legitimate security interests will need to be addressed. But what constitute 'legitimate' security interests is a matter of perspective. The security concern that Iran raises most frequently is the presence of 'imperialist' forces. Iran's demand for US, UK and French ships to leave the Gulf is intimately linked to its desire for a regional role. What Iran sees as a deserved role for itself in the region is seen by some of its neighbours as a hegemonic impulse, especially in light of the disruptive part Iran has played in events throughout the Middle East. For the Gulf states, concern about Iran getting the Bomb is almost matched by concern that the US and Iran will cut a deal behind their backs to give Iran more power at their expense. What is needed instead is a regional security structure that is inclusive and transparent.

Strengthening sanctions

Sharpening the contrast between the two paths open to Iran requires increasing the pressure in ways that impose real costs on Tehran decision-makers. It is not inconsistent to impose punitive sanctions while simultaneously seeking engagement. This kind of dual-track approach was well honed as part of the Cold War détente strategy. A tough dual approach could boost the chances of a more accommodating president replacing Ahmadinejad, who would probably gain less politically from his uncompromising policies if Iran was seen to be paying a real price for them.

The prospects for further meaningful sanctions by the Security Council were dim even before the deterioration of Western–Russian relations in the wake of Russia's incursion into Georgia in August 2008. Now, cooperation on new measures on Iran is far less likely. It is important nevertheless to sustain the sanctions already in place, as well as the framework of unity among the Security Council's permanent members. Although any new Security Council resolutions would be unlikely to impose attitude-changing costs, they would provide a political and legal basis for additional pressure from states willing to act on the issue. Short of adding new sanctions, one of the most effective steps the Security Council could take would be to establish an effective mechanism for monitoring the implementation of existing sanctions, using customs experts based in Dubai, the port where Iran has been most active in its efforts to circumvent sanctions through re-export arrangements.[11] Former US Treasury official Michael Jacobson reports that:

> The Dubai Deputy Chamber of Commerce and Industry estimated that in 2006 re-exports constituted 60% of the trade between [Dubai and Iran]. The deputy president of the Iranian

business council in Dubai bluntly assessed the sanctions' limitations, saying that they have 'virtually had no effect, to be honest.
If someone wants to move something – get it to Iran – it is easy
to be done.'[12]

The UAE re-exported about $8bn worth of goods to Iran in 2007, or
nearly a fifth of Iran's total imports.[13] The existing monitoring committee
for Security Council sanctions resolutions, comprised of representatives
of Belgium, Burkina Faso and Costa Rica, has no independent ability to
check implementation of provisions; it only receives reports from member
states about their national implementation measures. Although Council
members have discussed setting up a sanctions-monitoring body with
active verification responsibilities, the suggestion has not yet found strong
support.[14]

Whether additional sanctions are in the end adopted by the Security
Council, or, more likely, by concerned states acting outside the UN, it is
doubtful that new coercive measures alone would be effective in terms
of changing Iranian policy before the enrichment programme advances to
the point of giving Iran a latent weapons capability. However, sanctions
can help to keep that capability latent by denying Iran technology and
investment in industries that contribute to the programme and by creating negotiating leverage for insisting on conditions that would contribute
to keeping the programme limited and more transparent. Putting pressure on Iran in this way reinforces a point that cannot have been lost on
Iran's citizens – that their country cannot enjoy the respect, acceptance and
status it seeks as long as it continues to defy Security Council mandates
and pursue fissile-material technologies.

Sanctions also play an important deterrent role. Denying Iran the
policy benefits of its nuclear status by making it pay a price for defying
the Security Council sends an important signal to others who might wish
to follow the same route. This should be seen as part of a multifaceted
strategy for preventing a proliferation cascade in the Middle East. A key
part of such a strategy is to persuade states in the region that are interested
in nuclear power that fuel-cycle services are best obtained through the
international marketplace. In the event that the availability of foreign fuel-
cycle services backed by international guarantees does not persuade other
states in the region to forgo indigenous enrichment and reprocessing, the
responsibility for ensuring that nuclear energy in the Middle East does not
become a proliferation risk will have to be borne by outside powers. The
strategy should also include reassurances about Western security commit-

ments.[15] Any efforts to limit the expansion of enrichment and reprocessing technologies are unlikely to be successful, however, if Iran is seen as 'getting away with it'.

Containment and deterrence strategies

In the event that Iran does acquire a nuclear-weapons capability, containment and deterrence strategies will be critical to keeping Iran from crossing the line to production. Deterrence policies were employed effectively during the Cold War against far more powerful opponents, and there is reason to believe that such policies would be effective in forestalling the emergence of a nuclear-armed Iran. Modern Iran is no less rational than was the Soviet Union or Maoist China.[16] The case of China is instructive. When China was on the verge of acquiring nuclear weapons, the regime was widely seen as being heedless of human life and, therefore, not liable to be deterred from using such weapons to pose an existential threat to Taiwan. Yet, notwithstanding some very adverse consequences of China's nuclearisation, including the transfer of weapons designs to Pakistan (which later passed them to Libya), a weapons-capable China proved itself to be a rational actor that could in fact be deterred from using its nuclear arsenal. Similarly deterring Iran from using nuclear weapons would be more straightforward, however, than deterring the Islamic Republic from producing them. The latter is a new and more complicated application of deterrence theory.

Many Israelis claim that the Iranian regime is different, that, like a suicide bomber, it will be undeterrable, because of the apocalyptic belief of some of Ahmadinejad's supporters, and maybe even the president himself, that global chaos will hasten the return of the Madhi, a saviour-like figure central to Shia theology.[17] The historical record, however, suggests that when its national security is at stake, Iran behaves in a broadly rational manner. When Iraq launched missile attacks on Iranian cities in 1988 during the Iran–Iraq War, Ayatollah Khomeini, who had previously declared that he would not sign a ceasefire agreement with Saddam under any circumstances short of total Iraqi surrender, came to terms with the new situation and made compromises in order to end the war.[18] More recently, Iran showed restraint by not authorising Hizbullah to use long-distance rockets against Tel Aviv in the Lebanon War of summer 2006.[19]

Nuclear-deterrence theory is, unfortunately, not failsafe, particularly in transitional periods before adversaries have established robust command-and-control systems and communication channels with one another. For all their presumed rationality, the US and the USSR came close to engaging in nuclear war during the Cuban Missile Crisis in 1962, and India and Pakistan came perilously close in 2002 (and 1998). Iran seems to be more prone to miscalculation than those states, and less amenable to keeping open the communications channels required for stable deterrence. Mutual deterrence in the Middle East (between Israel and Iran) would become even less stable if Iran's example then led others to acquire nuclear-capable status.

Containment has been the US policy of choice on Iran since 1979. In its broad sense, the containment strategy today involves isolation and other means of denying Iran the ability to use a nuclear status to achieve the goals it seeks of Gulf hegemony and heightened prestige and status for the Islamic regime at home and abroad.[20] Containment entails de facto acquiescence in the existence of an opposing regime, but its purpose over the long term is to influence its behaviour and internal evolution by increasing the strains and contradictions under which its policies operate.[21] Vis-à-vis Iran, economic sanctions and financial isolation have been the principal means of executing the containment strategy. Iran, which has commercial dealings with 70 foreign partners, cannot be economically isolated any more than the Soviet Union could. But its spheres of economic activity can be significantly circumscribed. Political isolation cannot be complete either, especially in view of the Arab states' inclination to hedge their bets by alternating between containment and appeasement. Yet even imperfect isolation can deprive Iran of the benefits of national prestige, regional leadership and regime legitimisation it hopes will accrue from the nuclear programme.

A containment strategy based on isolation and deterrence has its drawbacks. Constraining investment in Iran's oil and gas sectors will not be sustainable in the long term, given increasing global demand and competition for energy supplies. Containment and deterrence by military encirclement could stimulate a regional arms race and a hardline response from Iran. According to Italian Middle East expert Riccardo Redaelli, Iran's reaction to the containment strategy over the past four years in particular has taken the form of what he calls the 'securitisation' of Iranian foreign policy and a radicalisation of Iranian domestic policy, whereby policymaking is held hostage to a radical interpretation of the security needs of the state. When Iranians feel they are under siege from without, Ahmadinejad and his fellow ultra-conservatives are better able to blame the US for the consequences of their leadership failures.[22]

If Redaelli is correct, and broad containment policies are found to be counterproductive, a more narrowly defined containment strategy must in any case be directed at constraining Iran's nuclear programme so that it does not cross the line to weaponisation. Notwithstanding differences over the broader policy of isolating Iran,[23] the elements of this more narrow construction of containment command widespread support. Tight export controls are aimed at preventing Iran from obtaining additional ring magnets, Fomblin oil, high-end vacuum pumps and other dual-use goods necessary for expanding its centrifuge programme. The extent to which export controls can impede the programme is subject to debate. Iran's demonstrated ability to expand its enrichment programme despite several years of export controls and intelligence scrutiny can be seen as an indication of the limits of such external controls. Where there is leakage, however, controls can be tightened. US-led containment policy today includes the PSI and the physical inspection of Iran-bound ships and aircraft authorised by UNSCR 1803. Western capitals undoubtedly have other, unpublicised tools that could contribute to delaying and limiting Iran's ability to produce enough HEU for a weapons capability. Containment measures should also include legal barriers to Iranian withdrawal from the NPT, such as a pre-emptive generic Security Council resolution that if a country found to be in safeguards non-compliance withdraws from the NPT, it forfeits the nuclear assets it acquired before withdrawal. Several such targeted containment tactics would be compatible with any fallback option and should be pursued regardless of which overall strategy is adopted towards Iran's nuclear programme. Fallback options designed to limit the size of Iran's enrichment programme are, of course, a kind of containment strategy in themselves.

Deterrence requires declaratory policies to let Iran know, by word and action, that the major powers would take whatever action was necessary to stop it from crossing the line to weapons acquisition, and that overwhelming force would be used against Iran in reprisal if it were to use or threaten to use nuclear weapons or provide such weapons or their components to others.[24] One reason that has been advanced for not issuing a declaratory warning to Tehran is that it might signal acceptance of a nuclear-armed Iran. This is reportedly why President Bush has not given a warning to Iran like the one he gave to North Korea in response to its nuclear test in October 2006, that 'transfer of nuclear weapons or material' to other countries or terrorist groups 'would be considered a grave threat to the United States'.[25] There would be less concern about appearing to acquiesce in an Iranian nuclear capability, however, if the red line cited was not the transfer of nuclear weapons but the possession of such weapons. The purpose of a declaratory policy is, after all, to strengthen the line between latent capability and weaponisation.

Deterring Iran from crossing the line to nuclear break-out will be a more viable strategic option to the extent that the line is made more visible. If the transatlantic allies ultimately decide to accept Iran's enrichment programme, among the minimal conditions for acceptance should be measures that would provide an easily detectable tripwire to signal break-out. A requirement that all LEU be stored outside the country might be one such tripwire condition. Minimal conditions should also include commitments by all the Security Council permanent members to impose harsh sanctions, including a full arms embargo, and to authorise use of force in the event of break-out.[26] Persuading Iran to accept the detectable tripwire conditions in the first instance and Russia and China to apply the penalties in the second may be impossible, however. Whatever conditions are specified, in practice, break-out is not likely to be a clearly visible, well-defined act with immediate consequences. Iran's modus operandi is likely to involve the accumulation of small transgressions, each of which individually would not necessarily sound the warning bell. If centrifuges were black-boxed, for example, Iran could justify opening one by citing safety reasons or the need to protect the stability of the rest of the cascade. Western powers would hardly bomb a plant or even shut it down over such an ill-defined transgression.[27] Additionally, Iran could use various ruses to delay the arrival of inspectors, buying time in order to be able to present the world with a fait accompli before Security Council members had time to act. In the event of clear break-out, Iran would be likely to try to evade severe penalties by trading off concessions on other priority issues for the West, such as counter-terrorism. It is not without reason that Iran has sought to discuss all issues concurrently by calling for 'comprehensive discussions'.[28]

Containment and deterrence strategies also include the reaffirmation of security commitments to Israel, Turkey and the Gulf states, deployment of theatre ballistic-missile-defence systems and the enhancement of other in-theatre capabilities. The US, the UK and France have in recent years been augmenting their military relationships in the region, strengthening the defensive capabilities of Iran's neighbours through joint training and other measures. Washington's $20bn arms-sale offer to Egypt, Jordan and the Gulf states in 2007 was intended, inter alia, to deter Iran and demonstrate America's resolve. Security reassurances from the major powers are both country-specific and regionwide, intended to underline that a nuclear-capable Iran will not be allowed to intimidate others.

As well as a credible threat of use of force if red lines are crossed, a successful deterrence strategy must include a corresponding reassurance to Iran's leaders that their country's sovereignty and security will not be threatened if red lines are observed.[29] The overall objective of the strategy is to influence Iran's strategic decision-making by reinforcing its reasons for stopping short of building nuclear weapons. All the elements devised to convince Iran's leadership to stop short are also part of the strategy to keep Iran from benefiting if it does acquire a nuclear bomb.[30]

In summary, offering a fallback option that legitimises enrichment in Iran is not the best way to reduce the proliferation risk. On one hand, the risks of diversion and clandestine operations would be lowered by options that increased IAEA inspection oversight and placed international engineers alongside Iranian operators. These non-proliferation benefits would be outweighed, however, by the increased potential for break-out that such schemes would entail as a result of their enhancement of Iran's access to technology and experience of production. Various technical fixes can be devised to try to detect and prevent cheating, but unless Iran made a fundamental decision to change its strategic objective, it would not accept restrictions on break-out opportunities or the level of intrusive inspections that would be required to quell the West's legitimate suspicions. Judging by its recent record, there is no reason to believe that Iran would accept and honour anything other than short-term limits with loopholes. Offering any deal that conceded legitimacy to the enrichment programme would also significantly weaken the West's negotiating position. Moreover, legitimising enrichment for Iran would contribute to the risk of a regional proliferation cascade by stimulating interest in enrichment elsewhere in the region. A dual policy of engagement and sanctions, with containment strategies targeted at limiting Iranian access to sensitive technologies and materials, is still the best way to test possibilities for Iranian cooperation while maintaining vigilance and controls to limit the nuclear-proliferation threat. If engagement fails, the sanctions strategy maintains a basis for long-term containment.[31]

NOTES

Introduction

[1] See for example Norman Podhoretz, 'Stopping Iran: Why the Case for Military Action Still Stands', *Commentary*, February 2008.

[2] Among those who have reached this or a similar conclusion are David Albright, Paul Brannan and Jacqueline Shire, in 'Can Military Strikes Destroy Iran's Gas Centrifuge Program? Probably Not', Institute for Science and International Security (ISIS), 7 August 2008, http://www.isis-online.org/publications/iran/Centrifuge_Manufacturing_7August2008.pdf; David Ignatius, in '"Bomb Bomb Iran"? Not Likely', *Washington Post*, 3 August 2008; Joseph Cirincione and Andrew Grotto, in 'Contain and Engage: A New Strategy for Resolving the Nuclear Crisis with Iran', Center for American Progress, March 2007; Paul R. Pillar, in 'What to Ask Before the Next War', *Washington Post*, 4 February 2007; Anatol Lieven, in 'Britain Must Act to Prevent an Attack on Iran', *Financial Times*, 6 July 2008; Anna Mulrine, in 'Why the Pentagon Thinks Attacking Iran is a Bad Idea', *US News and World Report*, 7 August 2008; Keith Crane, Rollie Lal and Jeffrey Martini, in 'Iran's Political, Demographic, and Economic Vulnerabilities', RAND, 2008; and David Kay, as paraphrased in Pamela Hess, 'Ex-Weapons Hunter: Iran 2–5 Years From Nuke Bomb', Associated Press, 1 October 2008.

[3] Bruno Tertrais made this observation at the IISS Global Strategic Review conference, 12–14 September 2008. Other non-nuclear-weapons states that have developed fissile-material technologies, for example Japan and Brazil, have not engaged in the kind of weapons-development work that Iran is assessed to have undertaken.

[4] Matthew Bunn, 'Constraining Iran's Nuclear Program: Assessing Options and Risks', presentation at Oak Ridge National Laboratory, Tennessee, 15 November 2007, http://belfercenter.ksg.harvard.edu/publication/17694/constraining_irans_nuclear_program.html.

Chapter One

1   Truck bombings on 23 October 1983 that killed 241 US servicemen and 58 French paratroopers were assessed by a US District Court judge to be the responsibility of Hizbullah acting in conjunction with Iranian agents, although Iran's culpability has not been firmly established.

2   In a 17 September 2005 address to the UN General Assembly, for example, President Mahmoud Ahmadinejad repeatedly asserted Iran's right to the nuclear fuel cycle.

3   For details of alleged weaponisation studies, see IAEA, 'Implementation of the NPT Safeguards Agreement and Relevant Provisions of Security Council Resolutions 1737 (2006) and 1747 (2007) in the Islamic Republic of Iran', GOV/2008/04, 22 February 2008, paras 35–41; and IAEA, 'Implementation of the NPT Safeguards Agreement and Relevant Provisions of Security Council Resolutions 1737 (2006), 1747 (2007) and 1803 (2008) in the Islamic Republic of Iran', GOV/2008/15, 26 May 2008, Annex.

4   Gareth Evans, 'The Right Nuclear Red Line', *Washington Post*, 5 December 2007; Trita Parsi, *Treacherous Triangle: The Secret Dealings of Israel, Iran and the United States* (New Haven, CT: Yale University Press, 2007), p. 269.

5   Bruno Tertrais, 'Has Iran Decided to Build the Bomb? Lessons from the French Experience', Carnegie Proliferation Analysis, 30 January 2007, http://www.carnegieendowment.org/publications/index.cfm?fa=view&id=18993.

6   For an insightful exposition of the muted debate in Iran about the value of nuclear weapons, see Shahram Chubin, *Iran's Nuclear Ambitions* (Washington DC: Carnegie Endowment for International Peace, 2006), pp. 28–36.

7   For a more detailed analysis of these points, see Mark Fitzpatrick, 'Assessing Iran's Nuclear Programme', *Survival*, vol. 48, no. 3, Autumn 2006, pp. 6–12.

8   IISS, *Iran's Strategic Weapons Programmes: A net assessment* (Abingdon: Routledge for the IISS, 2005), p. 46; IISS, *Nuclear Black Markets: Pakistan, A.Q. Khan and the rise of proliferation networks: A net assessment* (London: IISS, 2007), p. 67.

9   IAEA, 'Implementation of the NPT Safeguards Agreement in the Islamic Republic of Iran', GOV/2003/75, 10 November 2003. Paragraph 48 of the report summarises the violations.

10   IAEA, 'Implementation of the NPT Safeguards Agreement in the Islamic Republic of Iran: Resolution Adopted on 24 September 2005', GOV/2005/77, 24 September 2005.

11   Qatar was the only country to vote against the resolution.

12   Chubin, *Iran's Nuclear Ambitions*.

13   IAEA, GOV/2008/4, paras 11, 18.

14   IAEA, 'Implementation of the NPT Safeguards Agreement in the Islamic Republic of Iran', GOV/2006/15, 27 February 2006, para. 53.

15   Fitzpatrick, 'Assessing Iran's Nuclear Programme', p. 9.

16   IAEA, 'Communication Dated 27 August from the Permanent Mission of the Islamic Republic of Iran to the Agency Concerning the Text of the "Understandings of the Islamic Republic of Iran and the IAEA on the Modalities of Resolution of the Outstanding Issues"', INFCIRC/711, 27 August 2007.

17   IAEA, GOV/2008/15, Annex, p. 3.

18   *Ibid.*, Annex 1, p. 1.

19   Elaine Sciolino, 'Nuclear Aid by Russian to Iranians Suspected', *New York Times*, 10 October 2008.

20   IAEA, 'Implementation of the NPT Safeguards Agreement and Relevant Provisions of Security Council Resolutions 1737 (2006), 1747 (2007) and 1803 (2008) in the Islamic Republic of Iran', GOV/2008/38, 15 September 2008, paras 14–20.

21   Ze'ev Schiff, 'New Iranian Missiles Put Europe in Firing Range', *Haaretz*, 27

April 2006. The head of the intelligence branch of the Israel Defense Forces, Major-General Amos Yadlin, said in a speech in April 2006 that Iran had purchased 2,500km-range ground-to-ground missiles from North Korea.

22 Tests of the 1,900km rocket (which has a 50–100kg payload) in February and August 2008 failed, but each contributed to Iran's learning curve.

23 See for example Dinshaw Mistry, 'European Missile Defense: Assessing Iran's ICBM Capabilities', *Arms Control Today*, October 2007.

24 'Ukraine Admits Delivering Cruise Missiles to Iran, China', ITAR-TASS, 18 March 2005.

25 John Deutch, Ernest J. Moniz et al., 'The Future of Nuclear Power: An Interdisciplinary MIT Study', Massachusetts Institute of Technology, 2003. See also Sharon Squassoni, 'The Realities of Nuclear Expansion', Testimony before the US House of Representatives Select Committee on Energy Independence and Global Warming, 12 March 2008.

26 For a good summary of all 12 proposals, see Fiona Simpson, 'Reforming the Nuclear Fuel Cycle: Time is Running Out', *Arms Control Today*, September 2008.

27 Albert Wohlstetter, 'Spreading the Bomb Without Quite Breaking the Rules', *Foreign Policy*, no. 25, Winter 1976–1977.

28 In the late 1980s, Libya was able to obtain a detailed design of a reprocessing plant based on a German design from a source other than the A.Q. Khan network. IAEA, 'Implementation of the NPT Safeguards Agreement in the Socialist People's Libyan Arab Jamahiriya', GOV/2008/39, 12 September 2008, para. 31.

29 Iran has acknowledged that it conducted plutonium-separation experiments between 1988 and 1992.

30 Javad Zarif, 'An Unnecessary Crisis: Setting the Record Straight about Iran's Nuclear Program', advertisement published in the *New York Times*, 18

November 2005, http://www.un.int/iran/pressaffairs/pressreleases/1997/articles/1.html.

31 IAEA, GOV/2005/77, paras 1–2.

32 George Jahn, 'Russia Says it Won't Deliver Fuel to Iranian Reactor Without More Openness', Associated Press, 7 August 2007.

33 IAEA, GOV/2008/4, para. 54.

34 IAEA, INFCIRC/711. Iran's insistence appears to be based on the fact that the discussion of the alleged weaponisation studies is in a separate section of the work plan from the section that outlines efforts to address past outstanding issues.

35 See for example IAEA, 'Implementation of the NPT Safeguards Agreement and Relevant Provisions of Security Council Resolutions in the Islamic Republic of Iran', GOV/2007/22, 23 May 2007, para. 19.

36 The agency's right to such access is anticipated in the IAEA statute, Article XII.A.6. See Pierre Goldschmidt, 'IAEA Safeguards: Dealing Preventively with Non-Compliance', Harvard Belfer Center/Carnegie Endowment for International Peace, 12 July 2008, http://www.carnegieendowment.org/publications/index.cfm?fa=view&id=20308.

37 IAEA, 'Statement by the Board, 19 June 2003 (issued by the Chairwoman)', IAEA Media Advisory 2003/72, 19 June 2003.

38 IAEA, 'Implementation of the NPT Safeguards Agreement in the Islamic Republic of Iran', GOV/2003/40, 6 June 2003, paras 26, 32.

39 Text received privately from government official. The letter has not been made public.

40 IAEA, 'Statement by the Iranian Government and Visiting EU Foreign Ministers', 21 October 2003, http://www.iaea.org/NewsCenter/Focus/IaeaIran/statement_iran21102003.shtml.

41 IISS, *Iran's Strategic Weapons Programmes: A net assessment*, p. 20.

42 IAEA, 'Communication Dated 26 November 2004 Received from the Permanent Representatives of France,

Germany, the Islamic Republic of Iran and the United Kingdom Concerning the Agreement Signed in Paris on 15 November 2004', INFCIRC/637, 26 November 2004.

[43] Interview with European negotiator, November 2007.

[44] See for example Zarif, 'An Unnecessary Crisis: Setting the Record Straight about Iran's Nuclear Program'. Zarif claims that 'after massive pressure from the United States in the winter of 2005, the [E3] had conceded to unilaterally altering the Paris Agreement into solely an instrument of de-facto cessation of Iranian peaceful enrichment program, in violation of the letter and spirit of that Agreement'. In March 2005, Iran's chief negotiator, Hassan Rowhani, told a reporter that 'Every time the talks get serious the Europeans say they have to talk to the other side of the Atlantic.' Nazila Fathi, 'Iran Says It Won't Give Up Program to Enrich Uranium', *New York Times*, 6 March 2005.

[45] Interview with Rowhani by Mehdi Mohammadi, 'Nuclear Case from Beginning to End in Interview with Dr Hasan Rowhani (Part 1): We are Testing Europe', *Keyhan*, 26 July 2005, translated by the Foreign Broadcast Information Service.

[46] Interview with European negotiators, November 2007.

[47] Louis Charbonneau, 'Chirac Pushes EU to Drop Hard Line on Iran – Diplomats', Reuters, 13 April 2005.

[48] 'Europe "Rock-Solid" that Iran Cease Enrichment Ahead of New Talks', Agence France-Presse, 15 April 2005.

[49] IAEA, 'Communication Dated 8 August 2005 Received from the Resident Representatives of France, Germany and the United Kingdom to the Agency', INFCIRC/651, 8 August 2005.

[50] The six major parties involved in the Iran engagement strategy are formally known as the E3/EU+3, which reflects European primacy in the discussions with Iran, which are led by Solana and conducted on the basis of tactics and points for discussion largely drafted in London and Paris. In America, the group is commonly called the P5+1, a designation that emphasises the role of the permanent members of the Security Council.

[51] 'Elements of a Revised Proposal to Iran Made by the E3+3', 6 June 2006, attached as Annex II to UN Security Council Resolution 1747, 24 March 2007.

[52] This interpretation was offered by the Institute for Science and International Security (ISIS) in a cover note to the text of the 16 June 2008 that it circulated that day. The text of the offer is available on the ISIS website at http://www.isis-online.org/publications/iran/Diplomatic_Offer_16June2008.pdf, without the ISIS cover note. The author's conversations with officials in Washington and London in June 2008 confirmed that this interpretation is correct.

[53] Chubin, *Iran's Nuclear Ambitions*, p. 41.

[54] Tim Guldimann, 'Dealing with the Iranian Nuclear Programme', in Alexander Nikitin and Morten Bermer Maerli (eds), *Turning Priorities in Nuclear Arms Control and Non-Proliferation* (Amsterdam: IOS Press, 2008), p. 66.

Chapter Two

1. David Albright, Frans Berhout and William Walker, *Plutonium and Highly Enriched Uranium 1996: World Inventories, Capabilities and Policies* (New York: Oxford University Press, 1997), p. 359.

2. For examples of successful US diplomatic efforts to stop such sales, see Fitzpatrick, 'Lessons Learned from Iran's Pursuit of Nuclear Weapons', *Nonproliferation Review*, vol. 3, no. 3, November 2006, p. 534.

3. Warren Hoge, 'Iran Was Blocked From Buying Nuclear Materials at Least 75 Times, Group Says', *New York Times*, 16 November 2007.

4. Robert Joseph and Brendan Melley, 'Proliferation Pact Milestone', *Washington Times*, 28 May 2008.

5. Wade Boese, 'Interdiction Initiative Successes Assessed', *Arms Control Today*, vol. 38, no. 6, July–August 2008, p. 34.

6. Fitzpatrick, 'Lessons Learned from Iran's Pursuit of Nuclear Weapons', pp. 533–4.

7. Dafna Linzer, 'Iran is Judged 10 Years From Nuclear Bomb', *Washington Post*, 2 August 2005.

8. The author has no independent knowledge of any sabotage attempts other than what has been reported in open sources.

9. Martin Stoll, 'Atom-Affäre: CIA dealte mit Bern', *SonntagsZeitung*, 25 May 2008; Douglas Frantz and Catherine Collins, *The Nuclear Jihadist: The True Story of the Man Who Sold the World's Most Dangerous Secrets ... and How We Could Have Stopped Him* (New York: Twelve, 2007), p. 250: 'In one case, specialized vacuum pumps manufactured at the national weapons laboratory were identified and altered so they wouldn't work, before being shipped to Iran.'

10. William J. Broad and David E. Sanger, 'In Nuclear Net's Undoing, a Web of Shadowy Deals', *New York Times*, 25 August 2008.

11. Ian Black, 'Middle East: Death Sentence for Iranian Who Spied on Nuclear Project', *Guardian*, 1 July 2008.

12. James Risen, *State of War: The Secret History of the CIA and the Bush Administration* (London: Free Press, 2006), pp. 208–9.

13. Yossi Melman and Meir Javedanfar, *The Nuclear Sphinx of Tehran: Mahmoud Ahmadinejad and the State of Iran* (New York: Carroll & Graf Publishers, 2007), p. 199.

14. David Albright, Paul Brannan and Jacqueline Shire, 'Can Military Strikes Destroy Iran's Gas Centrifuge Program? Probably Not', Institute for Science and International Security, 7 August 2008. http://www.isis-online.org/publications/iran/Centrifuge_Manufacturing_7August2008.pdf.

15. Communication with European government official, September 2008.

16. Robert J. Einhorn, 'The U.S.–Russia Civil Nuclear Agreement', statement before the House Foreign Affairs Committee, 12 June 2008.

17. Chubin, *Iran's Nuclear Ambitions*, pp. 75–6; Karim Sadjadpour, *Reading Khamenei: The Word View of Iran's Most Powerful Leader*, Carnegie Endowment Report (Washington DC: Carnegie Endowment for International Peace, March 2008), p. 16; Riccardo Redaelli, 'Why Selective Engagement? Iranian and Western Interests are Closer Than You Think', Stanley Foundation Policy Analysis Brief, June 2008.

18. Scott Ritter, *Target Iran: The Truth About the White House's Plans for Regime Change* (London: Politico's, 2007), p. xxv.

19. This phrase was originally attributed to an unnamed senior British official. See 'Periscope', *Newsweek*, 19 August, 2002.

20. First reported without Bolton's name by Sonni Efron, 'Looking Past Baghdad to the Next Challenge', *Los Angeles Times*, 6 April 2003. Later attributed to Bolton by, inter alia, Joseph Cirincione, 'Failure in Iraq', Huffington Post, 5 May 2006.

21. IISS, *Nuclear Black Markets: Pakistan, A.Q. Khan and the rise of proliferation networks: A net assessment*, p. 97.

22 IAEA, INFCIRC/637.

23 'Council Common Position 2008/652/
CFSP of 7 August 2008 Amending
Common Position 2007/140/CFSP
Concerning Restrictive Measures Against
Iran', Official Journal of the European
Union, 8 August 2008, p. L 213/59.

24 'Australia Cenbank Imposes Sanctions on
Iran Entities', International Herald Tribune,
15 October 2008.

25 Also on 22 October, in a largely
symbolic sanction, the US used another
law (the Iran, North Korea and Syria
Nonproliferation Act) to bar the entire
IRGC from any US aid, contracts or arms
sales or other defence transfers.

26 For the October advisory, see http://www.
fatf-gafi.org/dataoecd/1/2/39481684.pdf,
for the February one, see http://www.
fatf-gafi.org/dataoecd/16/26/40181037.
pdf.

27 Deputy Assistant Secretary for Terrorist
Financing and Financial Crimes
Daniel Glaser, 'Between Feckless and
Reckless: U.S. Policy Options to Prevent
a Nuclear Iran', Testimony before the
House Committee on Foreign Affairs
Subcommittee on the Middle East and
South Asia and the Subcommittee on
Terrorism, Nonproliferation and Trade,
17 April 2008.

28 Daliah Merzaban, 'Iran Says Gulf Shields
its Banks from US Pressure', Middle East
Online, 6 February 2008.

29 Communication with French government
official, September 2008.

30 Steven Mufson and Robin Wright, 'Iran
Adapts to Economic Pressure', Washington
Post, 29 October 2007.

31 Michael Jacobson, 'Iran and the Road
Ahead', The Washington Institute for
Near East Policy, PolicyWatch no. 1350,
6 March 2008.

32 Patrick Seale, 'Is Undermining Iran an
Arab or European Interest?', Middle East
Online, 19 May 2008.

33 Charles Bremner, 'Iran Isolation Grows
as France's Total Cancels $10bn South
Pars Gas Field Project', The Times, 11 July
2008.

34 Mark Landler, 'Germany's Commercial
Ties with Iran Prove Hard to Cut', New
York Times, 21 September 2007.

35 Assaf Uni and Barak Ravid, 'Despite
Sanctions, German Firm Closes 100m Euro
Deal with Iran', Haaretz, 31 July 2008.

36 'Russia's Gazprom Looks to Expand
Business with Iran', Reuters, 13 July
2008.

37 Kenneth Katzman, 'The Iran Sanctions
Act (ISA)', Congressional Research
Service Report for Congress, 12 October
2007, p. 6.

38 Matthew Levitt, 'Making Iran Feel the
Pain', Wall Street Journal, 2 July 2007.

39 Glaser, 'Between Feckless and Reckless:
U.S. Policy Options to Prevent a Nuclear
Iran'.

40 Jim Hoagland, 'Jitters over Iran',
Washington Post, 13 July 2008.

41 Gordon Brown, 'Lord Mayor's Banquet
Speech', 12 November 2007.

42 Adam Zagorin, 'Still Trying to Squeeze
Iran', Time, 31 January 2008.

43 Brian Radzinsky, 'States Divest From
Businesses Tied to Iran', Arms Control
Today, July–August 2008.

44 David Miliband, 'Iran: Export Credit
Guarantees', Daily Hansard Written
Answers 30 June 2008, Column 674W.

45 Communication with Italian Foreign
Ministry official, October 2008.

46 Mufson and Wright, 'Iran Adapts to
Economic Pressure'.

47 Timothy Garton Ash, 'Facing Disaster in
Iran, Europe Must Finally Make the Hard
Choices', Guardian, 1 November 2007.

48 Britain Israel Communications and
Research Centre, 'BICOM Analysis:
Sanctions Policy Briefing Note', 10 August
2008.

49 Levitt, 'Making Iran Feel the Pain'.

50 In December 2005, Russia agreed to sell
TOR-M1 anti-aircraft missile systems to
Iran at an estimated cost of $700m. Other
deals between 2001 and 2005 totalled an
estimated $400m. In December 2007, Iran
claimed to have signed a contract with
Russia for supply of S-300 (SA-10) air-
defence systems at an undisclosed price,

see Doug Richardson, 'Iran May Have Lined up S-300 SAM Systems', *Jane's Industry Quarterly*, 9 January 2008.

51 Ashton B. Carter and William J. Perry, 'Plan B for Iran: What if Nuclear Diplomacy Fails?', report of the Preventive Defense Project, 10 September 2006.

52 According to former Director of the German–Iranian Chamber of Commerce Michael Tockuss, around two-thirds of Iran's industry is equipped to a significant degree with German-origin machinery. Christoph Elflein, 'Wirtschaft drohen Milliardenverluste', *Focus*, 13 February 2006.

53 Yossi Sarid, 'Real Sanctions Will Cool Off the Ayatollahs', http://www.bitterlemons-international.org, 3 April 2008.

54 Dennis Ross, 'Choices and Strategies for Dealing with Iran', Testimony to the Senate Homeland Security and Governmental Affairs Subcommittee on Federal Financial Management, Government Information, Federal Services, and International Security, 24 April 2008.

55 Matthew Lee, 'Analysis: US and Iran Appear on Collision Course', Associated Press, 9 July 2008.

56 'Iran: US, Israel Spread Iranophobia', Fars News Agency, 18 July 2008.

57 Jim Walsh, 'Addressing Iran's Nuclear Ambitions', Testimony to the Senate Homeland Security and Governmental Affairs Subcommittee on Federal Financial Management, Government Information, Federal Services, and International Security, 24 April 2008, p. 6.

58 William Luers, Thomas R. Pickering and Jim Walsh, 'A Solution for the US–Iran Nuclear Standoff', *New York Review of Books*, vol. 55, no. 4, 20 March 2008.

59 Albright, Shire and Brannan, 'IAEA Report on Iran: Centrifuge Operation Significantly Improving; Gridlock on Alleged Weaponization Issues'.

60 IAEA, 'Implementation of the NPT Safeguards Agreement and Relevant Provisions of Security Council Resolutions 1737 (2006), 1747 (2007), 1803 (2008) and 1835 (2008) in the Islamic Republic of Iran', GOV/2008/59, para. 2.

61 Albright, Shire and Brannan, 'IAEA Report on Iran: Centrifuge Operation Significantly Improving; Gridlock on Alleged Weaponization Issues'. As Albright notes, for Iran, it could take between 1,000kg and 1,700kg of LEU to make one bomb's worth of HEU.

62 '15th Ministerial Conference of the Non-Aligned Movement, Statement on the Islamic Republic of Iran's Nuclear Issue', NAM 2008/Doc.3/Rev.1, para. 2.

63 Fredrik Dahl, 'Iran Tells Developing States to Fight UN "Bias"', Reuters, 29 July 2008, http://www.reuters.com/article/worldNews/idUSL920861420080729.

64 Nazila Fathi and Michael Slackman, 'Iran's President Criticized Over Nuclear Issue', *New York Times*, 18 January 2007.

65 Ali Akbar Dareini, 'Iran's Ex-Nuke Negotiator Lambastes Ahmadinejad's International Dealings and Economic Policies', Associated Press, published in *International Herald Tribune*, 10 October 2007.

66 'Iran's Ex-Nuke Negotiator Slams Ahmadinejad on Key Policies', Associated Press, published in *International Herald Tribune*, 11 December 2007.

67 See Borzou Daragahi and Ramin Mostaghim, 'Iran Sanctions Ripple Past Those in Power', *Los Angeles Times*, 20 January 2008.

68 Walsh, 'Addressing Iran's Nuclear Ambitions', p. 8.

69 Fathi, 'A President's Defender Keeps His Distance', *New York Times*, 8 January 2008.

70 Reported in Seyyed Abedin Nureddini, 'Do Not Break This Taboo', published in an Iranian newspaper, 20 May 2008 [in Persian], available from BBC Monitoring (newspaper unspecified).

71 William J. Burns, 'US Policy Toward Iran', Opening Statement before the House Foreign Affairs Committee, 9 July 2008.

72 'Iran's Unemployment Falls to 10.3 Percent', Fars News Agency, 1 April 2008.

73 Volker Perthes, 'Of Trust and Security: The Challenge of Iran', in Volker Perthes, Ray

Takeyh and Hitoshi Tanaka, *Engaging Iran and Building Peace in the Persian Gulf Region* (Washington DC: Trilateral Commission, 2008), Task Force Report no. 62, p. 54.

[74] Burns, 'US Policy Toward Iran'.

[75] Stanley Reed, 'Surprise: Oil Woes in Iran', *Business Week*, 30 November 2006.

[76] US Government Accountability Office, 'Iran Sanctions: Impact in Furthering U.S. Objectives Is Unclear and Should be Reviewed', GAO-08-58, December 2007.

[77] An October 2008 report from Deutsche Bank Global Markets Research found that $95 a barrel is the break-even price for Iran. See 'Measuring 'Cheap' Oil', *Oil & Gas Journal*, vol. 106, issue 39, 20 October 2008.

[78] Laurent Zecchini, 'L'embargo qui fait peur à Tehran', *Le Monde*, 20 January 2007.

[79] Daragahi and Mostaghim, 'Iran Sanctions Ripple Past Those in Power'.

[80] As privately reported to a Western ambassador to Iran, April 2008.

[81] John Ward Anderson, 'E.U. Backs Sanctions on Iran, Freezes Bank Assets', *Washington Post*, 24 June 2008.

[82] Dahl, 'Iran Says New Sanctions will Not Hurt Economy', Reuters, 5 March 2008.

[83] Merzaban, 'Iran Says Gulf Shields its Banks from U.S. Pressure'.

[84] Mossad Director Meir Dagan told a Knesset committee in December 2006 that 'such a concept [as the point of no return] does not exist'. Ben Aluf and Gideon Alon, 'Mossad Chief: Iran Will Not Get Nuclear Bomb Before 2009', *Haaretz*, 19 December 2006.

[85] Emily B. Landau, 'Iran's Nuclear Advances: The Politics of Playing with Time', Institute for National Security Studies (Israel) Strategic Assessment, vol. 10, no. 1, June 2007, http://www.inss.org.il/publications.php?cat=25&incat=&read=19.

[86] For an insightful analysis of how intelligence estimates have been used as part of an Israeli propaganda effort, see Reuven Pedatzur, 'The Iranian Nuclear Threat and the Israeli Options', *Contemporary Security Policy*, vol. 28, no. 3, December 2007.

[87] Thomas B. Cochran, 'Adequacy of IAEA's Safeguards for Achieving Timely Detection', in Henry D. Sokolski (ed.), *Falling Behind: International Scrutiny of the Peaceful Atom* (Carlisle, PA: Strategic Studies Institute, February 2008), p. 137.

[88] Mark Hibbs, 'Bellows, Bearing Stress Led Japan to Abandon Squat Centrifuges', *Nuclear Fuel*, 4 June 2007.

[89] IAEA, GOV/2008/15, para. 2.

[90] Although 54,000 machines is the most commonly stated goal, in April 2006, Atomic Energy Organisation of Iran Director Gholam-Reza Aqazadeh said that the Natanz plant would house 48,000 centrifuges.

[91] IISS, *Iran's Strategic Weapons Programmes: A net assessment*, pp. 54, 56.

[92] David Albright and Jacqueline Shire, 'A Witches' Brew? Evaluating Iran's Uranium-Enrichment Progress', *Arms Control Today*, November 2007.

[93] 'Nuclear Iran – How Close is It?', IISS *Strategic Comments*, vol. 13, no. 7, 27 September 2007; Albright and Shire, 'A Witches' Brew? Evaluating Iran's Uranium-Enrichment Progress'.

[94] IAEA, 'Implementation of the NPT Safeguards Agreement in the Islamic Republic of Iran', GOV/2004/83, 15 November 2004, para. 45.

[95] Albright and Shire, 'A Witches' Brew? Evaluating Iran's Uranium-Enrichment Progress'.

[96] Communications with David Albright and Jacqueline Shire, August and September 2008.

[97] Richard L. Garwin, 'When Could Iran Deliver a Nuclear Weapon?', *Bulletin of the Atomic Scientists*, 18 January 2008.

[98] Thomas B. Cochran and Christopher E. Paine, 'The Amount of Plutonium and Highly-Enriched Uranium Needed for Pure Fission Nuclear Weapons', Natural Resources Defense Council, 13 April 1995.

[99] This represents the theoretical operating time needed for a 3,000-machine facility to produce 25kg of 93% HEU. A 50,000-machine facility could produce weapons-grade HEU from LEU stock in

two to three days. IISS, *Iran's Strategic Weapons Programme: A net assessment*, p. 55.

100   Although batch processing – running the LEU through the same cascade configuration multiple times – can produce HEU, to do so efficiently as part of an ongoing programme, reconfiguration of the cascades and piping or, alternatively, construction of an additional set of centrifuge modules is required. Reconfiguring a plant like Natanz for HEU production would not be easy for a state without experience in vacuum technologies, but some sources have reported that Iran acquired information from the Khan network on how to do this. See Albright and Shire, 'A Witches' Brew? Evaluating Iran's Uranium-Enrichment Progress'.

101   Anna M. Pluta and Peter D. Zimmerman, 'Nuclear Terrorism: A Disheartening Dissent', *Survival*, vol. 48, no. 2, Summer 2006, p. 64.

102   Jafar Dhia Jafar and Numan Al-Niaimi, *Iraqi Weapons Mass Destruction (WMD): Fact and Fiction* (Beirut: Centre for Arab Unity Studies, May 2005) [in Arabic], http://www.caus.org.lb/Home/publication_popup.php?ID=3528&h=1.

103   'On the Possibility of Developing Nuclear Weapons Domestically', *Sankei Shimbun*,

25 December 2006 [in Japanese]. For an English summary of the main points of this article, see 'How Long Would it Take Japan?', 26 December 2006, http://www.armscontrolwonk.com/1336/how-long-would-it-take-japan. Several Western experts have suggested that it would take Japan only six months to produce a nuclear weapon, but this estimate has not been subject to rigorous analysis. For an example of such estimates, see Frank Barnaby and Shaun Burnie, 'Thinking the Unthinkable: Japanese Nuclear Power and Proliferation in East Asia', *Japan Focus*, 8 September 2005.

104   Michael Hayden, 'The CIA's Counterproliferation Efforts', address to the Los Angeles World Affairs Council, 16 September 2008.

105   Albright, 'Swiss Smugglers Had Advanced Nuclear Weapons Designs', Institute for Science and International Security, 16 June 2008.

106   Frantz and Collins, *The Nuclear Jihadist: The True Story of the Man Who Sold the World's Most Dangerous Secret ... and How We Could Have Stopped Him*, p. 348.

107   Albright, 'Swiss Smugglers Had Advanced Nuclear Weapons Designs', p. 1.

108   *Ibid.*

Chapter Three

1   Linzer, 'IAEA Head Waits to Issue Iran Verdict', *Washington Post*, 1 March 2005.

2   William J. Broad, 'The Thin Line Between Civilian and Military Nuclear Programs', *New York Times*, 5 December 2007.

3   Evans, 'The Right Nuclear Red Line'.

4   See 'Report of the Commission to Assess the Ballistic Missile Threat to the United States: Executive Summary', 15 July 1998, II.C.4b, http://www.fas.org/irp/threat/missile/rumsfeld/toc.htm.

5   Walsh, 'Addressing Iran's Nuclear Ambitions'.

6   David Sanger and Thom Shanker, 'Washington Sees an Opportunity on Iran', *New York Times*, 27 September 2007.

7   Luers, Pickering and Walsh, 'A Solution for the US–Iran Nuclear Standoff'.

8   International Crisis Group, 'Iran: Is there a Way Out of the Nuclear Impasse?', Middle East Report no. 51, 23 February 2006.

9   Evans, 'The Iran Nuclear Problem: The Way Forward', presentation to the 'International Seminar on Iran's Nuclear Program and the IAEA Director-General's

Report', School of International Relations, Ministry of Foreign Affairs, Tehran, 22 November 2007.

[10] Sciolino, 'Russia Plan for Iran Upsets U.S. and Europe', *New York Times*, 7 March 2006.

[11] International management of Iran's nuclear sites was first briefly raised as a possibility by the International Crisis Group in 'Dealing with Iran's Nuclear Program', Middle East Report no. 18, 27 October 2003. Among other early advocates was Maurizio Martellini, Secretary-General of the Italy-based security think tank Landau Network-Centro Volta, who in February 2006 floated the idea of small-scale uranium-enrichment research activities in Iran under the auspices of an international consortium or as a multilateral joint venture. Others who argue that multinational-consortium ownership offers the best option for minimising the proliferation risk include Jason Blackstock and Manjana Milkoreit, 'Understanding the Iranian Nuclear Equation', *Journal of Public and International Affairs*, vol. 18, Spring 2007.

[12] See Geoffrey Forden and John Thomson, 'A Shared Solution to the Iran Nuclear Stand-Off', *Financial Times*, 20 February 2006. For their full proposal, see Forden and Thomson, 'Iran as a Pioneer Case for Multilateral Nuclear Arrangements', Science, Technology and Global Security Working Group, Massachusetts Institute of Technology, 2006 (revised 2007).

[13] Luers, Pickering and Walsh, 'A Solution for the US–Iran Nuclear Standoff'.

[14] Bunn, 'Constraining Iran's Nuclear Program: Assessing Options and Risks'.

[15] For a thorough elaboration of Iran's position, see Zarif, 'An Unnecessary Crisis: Setting the Record Straight about Iran's Nuclear Program'.

[16] 'Iran: Nuclear Time-Out, Not Suspension', Press TV (Iranian news agency), 26 July 2007.

[17] 'Une heure avec le président iranien, Mahmoud Ahmadinejad', *Le Monde*, 5 February 2008.

[18] Julian Borger, 'Iran Calls for Uranium Enrichment on its Soil, with the World's Help', *Guardian*, 23 May 2008.

[19] Gary Samore, 'Policy Options Paper: Iran', unpublished draft report, Council on Foreign Relations, 30 January 2008.

[20] On occasion, Iranian officials have seemed to suggest this, but with deliberate ambiguity. Atomic Energy Organisation of Iran Deputy Director Mohammad Saeedi told the France Info radio station in 2006 that a solution to the nuclear issue might be a consortium arrangement with France to enrich uranium in Iran, which would enable France to 'control in a tangible way our enrichment activities'. 'Iran Pushes France Nuclear Deal', BBC News Online, 2 October 2006. More recently, US Senator Dianne Feinstein came away from informal talks involving former Iranian Ambassador to the UN Javad Zarif with the impression that Iran might be prepared to submit its facilities to international monitoring. Feinstein reported that 'some of the Iranian side thought that Iranian leadership – namely the Supreme Leader – might be open to the idea of an "on-the-ground 24/7 international consortium" to manage and monitor all aspects of nuclear activity. There was agreement that Iran might agree to this monitoring – as long as there was an openness on the part of the United States to discuss other issues as well.' Dianne Feinstein, 'Breaking the US–Iran Stalemate', speech to the National Iranian American Council, 8 April 2008.

[21] See for example Walsh, 'Addressing Iran's Nuclear Ambitions', p. 12.

[22] Massimo Calabresi, 'U.S. and Iran: A One-Sided Negotiation', *Time*, 21 July 2008.

[23] Former UK ambassador to the IAEA Peter Jenkins made this point to an IISS workshop, September 2008.

[24] Fitzpatrick, 'Can Iran's Nuclear Capability Be Kept Latent?', *Survival*, vol. 29, no. 1, Spring 2007, p. 50.

[25] Rowhani, 'Beyond the Challenges Facing Iran and the IAEA Concerning the Nuclear Dossier', *Rahbord*, 30 September 2005 [in Persian], translated in 2006 by the Foreign

Broadcast Information Service (FBIS-IAP20060113336001) and downloadable from Arms Control Wonk.com, www.armscontrolwonk.com/file_download/30.

26 WorldPublicOpinion.org, 'Public Opinion in Iran: With Comparisons to American Public Opinion', 7 April 2008.

27 Sadjadpour, *Reading Khamenei: The World View of Iran's Most Powerful Leader*, pp. 15–16. Khamenei reiterated his position on 30 July 2008: 'Taking one step back against arrogant [powers] will lead to them to take one step forward'. Ian Black, 'Iran Vows to Stay on "Nuclear Path" as UN Deadline Looms', *Guardian*, 31 July 2008.

28 'Iran Rejects Intrusive Nuclear Inspections as Unfair in View of Israel', Associated Press, published in *International Herald Tribune*, 5 May 2008.

29 Zarif, 'An Unnecessary Crisis: Setting the Record Straight about Iran's Nuclear Program'.

30 In 2003, Iran was the last state with significant nuclear activities to accept the modified Code 3.1 of the Subsidiary Arrangements to the Safeguards Agreement, which replaced what had been a requirement to submit design information for new facilities 'normally not later than 180 days before the facility is scheduled to receive nuclear material for the first time'. In March 2007, in response to UNSCR 1747, Iran unilaterally reverted to the earlier form of Code 3.1. As the IAEA has pointed out (see IAEA, GOV/2007/22, para. 14), agreed subsidiary arrangements cannot be modified unilaterally.

31 See for example Evans, 'The Right Nuclear Red Line'; Flynt Leverett and Hillary Mann Leverett, 'How to Defuse Iran', *New York Times*, 11 December 2007; and Ray Takeyh, 'Shaping a Nuclear Iran', *Washington Post*, 18 May 2008. Henry Kissinger came close to saying the same when he remarked in a May 2008 interview that 'The challenge is to find a formula for resolving the Iran nuclear issue that allows for effective supervision and control acceptable to the international community'. Stephen Graubard, 'Lunch with the FT: Henry Kissinger', *Financial Times*, 23 May 2008.

32 'Reinforcing the Global Nuclear Order for Peace and Prosperity: The Role of the IAEA to 2020 and Beyond' report prepared by an independent commission at the request of the Director General of the International Atomic Energy Agency, May 2008. The commission suggested that ultimately all IAEA member states should accept the IAEA's right 'to access sites and information related to nuclear material production technologies (such as centrifuge manufacturing facilities) and to nuclear weaponization activities, as well as the Agency's right to private interviews with individuals who may know about such activities'. The commission's call for universal application of an 'Additional Protocol Plus' was met with immediate disfavour by many developing countries, which are loath to accept yet more non-proliferation obligations while states that possess nuclear weapons face no obligation to take disarmament steps.

33 IAEA, 'Implementation of the NPT Safeguards Agreement in the Islamic Republic of Iran', GOV/2005/67, 2 September 2005. For the subsequent Board endorsement, see 'Implementation of the NPT Safeguards Agreement in the Islamic Republic of Iran: Resolution Adopted on 4 February 2006', GOV/2006/14.

34 Goldschmidt, 'IAEA Safeguards: Dealing Preventively with Non-Compliance'.

35 See quotations and references in Michael Hirsh, 'Iran Has a Message. Are We Listening?', *Washington Post*, July 2007; Parsi, *Treacherous Triangle: The Secret Dealings of Israel, Iran and the United States*; and Kassem Ja'afar, 'Bombing Iran or Living with Iran's Bomb? The Price of Military Action, the Consequences of Inaction', Transatlantic Institute, July 2008.

36 Luers, Pickering and Walsh, 'A Solution for the US–Iran Nuclear Standoff'; Walsh, 'Addressing Iran's Nuclear Ambitions'.

37 Walsh, 'Addressing Iran's Nuclear Ambitions'.

38 Debate on this point would benefit from a technical review informed by classified

information about state-of-the-art and over-the-horizon detection and environmental sample analysis techniques.

39 Fitzpatrick, 'Can Iran's Nuclear Capability Be Kept Latent?', pp. 53–4.

40 Forden and Thomson, 'A Shared Solution to the Iran Nuclear Stand-off'. See also Walsh, 'Addressing Iran's Nuclear Ambitions', p. 17.

41 Blackstock and Milkoreit, 'Uranium Enrichment on Iranian Soil: Evaluating and Minimizing the Risks', discussion paper, Belfer Center, Harvard Kennedy School (forthcoming).

42 Luers, Pickering and Walsh, 'A Solution for the US–Iran Nuclear Standoff'; Bunn, 'Constraining Iran's Nuclear Program: Assessing Options and Risks'.

43 The most infamous case of Iranian hostage-taking is that of the 52 US diplomats held by Iranian student militants in the US embassy in Tehran from November 1979 to January 1981. The most recent example is that of 15 British naval personnel held hostage for 13 days by the Iranian military in spring 2007.

44 This idea is put forward in Luers, Pickering and Walsh, 'A Solution for the US–Iran Nuclear Standoff'.

45 Blackstock and Milkoreit, 'Understanding the Iranian Nuclear Equation'.

46 In a speech on 14 December 2001, Rafsanjani said, 'If one day the Islamic world is also equipped with weapons like those that Israel possesses now, then the imperialists' strategy will reach a standstill because the use of even one nuclear bomb inside Israel will destroy everything [in Israel]. [But] it will only harm the Islamic world.'

47 IISS, *Nuclear Programmes in the Middle East: In the shadow of Iran* (London: IISS, 2008), pp. 7–9.

48 *Ibid.*, pp. 42–7.

49 Luers, Pickering and Walsh, 'A Solution for the US–Iran Nuclear Standoff'.

50 Fitzpatrick, 'Can Iran's Nuclear Capability Be Kept Latent?', p. 53.

51 Goldschmidt, 'Rule of Law, Politics and Nuclear Nonproliferation', presentation to the Ecole Internationale de Droit Nucléaire, University of Montpellier, France, 2007, published 7 November 2007; http://www.carnegieendowment.org/publications/index.cfm?fa=view&id=19564.

52 As Jim Walsh acknowledges, in Walsh, 'Addressing Iran's Nuclear Ambitions'.

Conclusion

1 'Nuclear Iran – How Close is It?'.

2 George Perkovich, 'Iran Says "No" – Now What?', Carnegie Endowment for International Peace, Policy Brief no. 63, September 2008.

3 Kelly Campbell, 'Analyzing Iran's Domestic Political Landscape', United States Institute of Peace briefing, May 2008.

4 For an example of this view, see Flynt Leverett, 'Dealing with Tehran: Assessing U.S. Diplomatic Options Toward Iran', Century Foundation Report, December 2006.

5 Andrea Claudia Hoffmann, 'Wir spielen keine Spielchen', *Focus* no. 32, 6 August 2007.

6 Mehdi Mohammadi, 'A Failed Mark in the Imperialists' "Report Card"', *Keyhan* website, 1 July 2008, translated by BBC Monitoring.

7 Ray Takeyh, 'Time for Détente with Iran', *Foreign Affairs*, March–April 2007.

8 Presentation at IISS, London, October 2007.

9 IISS, *Iran's Strategic Weapons Programmes: A net assessment*, p. 22.

10 Parsi, *Treacherous Triangle: The Secret Dealings of Israel, Iran and the United States*, pp. 243–9 and 341–6.

11 In an attempt to thwart these efforts, the UAE in 2008 sharply reduced the number of business licences and work visas it

granted to Iranian citizens. See Farah Stockman, 'U.S. Sanctions Hit Iranian Entrepreneurs in Dubai', *Boston Globe*, 16 September 2008.

[12] Jacobson, 'Putting the Squeeze on Iran', *Guardian*, 22 July 2008.

[13] Dareini, 'Sanctions Slow Iran's Trade, But Not Stop', Associated Press, 18 August 2008.

[14] Herb Keinon, 'UN Must Monitor Sanctions Compliance', *Jerusalem Post*, 28 October 2008.

[15] See IISS, *Nuclear Programmes in the Middle East: In the shadow of Iran*, pp. 161–2.

[16] Among those who have emphasised this point are former US National Security Advisor Zbigniew Brzezinski, interviewed by the Center for Strategic And International Studies, 'CSIS-Schieffer Dialogue: Opening Steps for a Diplomatic Path Between the U.S. And Iran', 22 July 2008; Gideon Rose, in 'Revisiting Iran', *National Interest*, March–April 2007; and Pillar, in 'What to Ask Before the Next War'.

[17] For examples of this view, see 'Explaining Iran', editorial, *Jerusalem Post*, 3 November 2007; Noah Feldman, 'Islam, Terror and the Second Nuclear Age', *New York Times Magazine*, 29 October 2006.

[18] Pedatzur, 'The Iranian Nuclear Threat and the Israeli Options', p. 534; Parsi, 'The Iranian Challenge', *The Nation*, 1 November 2007.

[19] Parsi, 'The Iranian Challenge'.

[20] Lewis A. Dunn, 'After Iranian Acquisition, What? Containing the Dangers of a Proliferating Middle East', unpublished paper prepared for the William S. Cohen Center, University of Maine and the National Defense University, 9 July 2007.

[21] Richard N. Haass, 'Regime Change and its Limits', *Foreign Affairs*, July–August 2005.

[22] Redaelli, 'Why Selective Engagement? Iranian and Western Interests are Closer Than You Think'.

[23] Among other scholars who argue for détente over containment, see Takeyh, 'Time for Détente with Iran'; Parsi,

Treacherous Triangle: The Secret Dealings of Israel, Iran and the United States; and Michael McFaul, Abbas Milani and Larry Diamond, 'A Win–Win U.S. Strategy for Dealing with Iran', *Washington Quarterly*, vol. 30, no. 1, Winter 2006–7.

[24] For discussion of such declaratory policies, see for example Haass, 'Regime Change and its Limits'; and Charles Krauthammer, 'The Holocaust Declaration', *Washington Post*, 11 April 2008.

[25] Sanger and Shanker, 'U.S. Rethinks Atomic Deterrence in Terror Age', *International Herald Tribune*, 9 May 2007.

[26] At an IISS workshop on Iran in Geneva on 15 September 2008, Jean-Louis Gergorin, discussing the need to enhance the visibility of break-out, suggested what would perhaps be more achievable conditions (but which, in the author's view, would not be sufficient): a requirement to convert all LEU to fuel assemblies, accompanied by an only implicit threat of use of force in case of violation.

[27] James Acton offered this example at a workshop on disarmament and the nuclear industry at the IISS, London, 5 September 2008.

[28] The author is indebted to Ariel Levite for suggesting this point.

[29] Patrick Clawson, 'Deterrence and Regime Change', in Patrick Clawson and Michael Eisenstadt (eds), *Deterring the Ayatollahs: Complications in Applying Cold War Strategy to Iran* (Washington DC: Washington Institute for Near East Policy, July 2007), Policy Focus no. 72. Jeffrey Lewis also emphasises this point in his companion article in the same publication, 'Assumptions Underlying the Debate on Deterring Emerging Nuclear States'.

[30] Dunn, 'After Iranian Acquisition, What? Containing the Dangers of a Proliferating Middle East'.

[31] Cirincione and Grotto, 'Contain and Engage: A New Strategy for Resolving the Nuclear Crisis with Iran', p. 35.

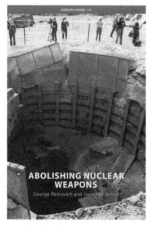
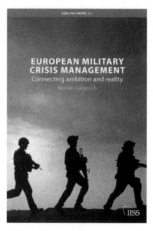
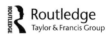